Comments on **Psoriasis at your fingertips** *from readers*

'I am sure this book will be very well received.'
   Dr Mary Judge, Consultant Dermatologist, Royal Bolton Hospital

'For those who may have just been diagnosed as having psoriasis, this book will explain much about the disease, its symptoms and treatments. It has medical remedies for keeping your skin in the best possible condition, as well as exploring the psychological effects the disease can have on the sufferer.'
   John Bevan, Farnham

Here it is: all you wanted to know but didn't like to ask your busy GP; all you were told but didn't quite grasp, or forgot as soon as you left the consulting room. Relax, and absorb the answers in comfort.
   Valerie Elliston, Colchester

D0182932

Psoriasis at your fingertips

THE COMPREHENSIVE AND MEDICALLY ACCURATE MANUAL ON MANAGING PSORIASIS

Tim Mitchell   MB ChB, MRCGP, DRCOG, DPD
GP in inner city Bristol; founder member and secretary of the Primary Care Dermatology Society; Specialist adviser to the All Party Parliamentary Group on Skin; member of the International Psoriasis Board

and

Rebecca Penzer   RGN, BSc (Hons), PGDip Advanced Practice, PGDip Professional Education
Specialist dermatology nurse, formerly at QualityCare, Wellingborough

CLASS PUBLISHING · LONDON

The rights of Tim Mitchell and Rebecca Penzer to be identified as the authors
of this work have been asserted by them in accordance with the Copyright,
Designs and Patents Act 1988

Printing history
First published 2000

The authors and publishers welcome feedback from the users of this book.
Please contact the publishers.
**Class Publishing (London) Ltd, Barb House, Barb Mews, London W6 7PA
Telephone: 020 7371 2119; Fax 020 7371 2878 [International +4420]**

A CIP catalogue record for this book is available from the British Library.

ISBN 1 872362 99 0

Edited by Gillian Clarke

Designed by Wendy Bann

Cartoons by Jane Taylor

Index by Valerie Elliston

Typeset by Sally Brock, High Wycombe, Buckinghamshire

Produced by Landmark Production Consultants Ltd, Princes Risborough

Printed and bound in Finland by WS Bookwell, Juva

Contents

Acknowledgements

We are grateful to all the people who have helped in the production of this book, and in particular we thank the following for their contributions and support:

Professor Andrew Finlay, Professor of Dermatology in Cardiff, for writing the Foreword;

Dr Mary Judge, Consultant Dermatologist in Manchester, for reviewing the manuscript and commenting on various drafts;

the Psoriasis Association, especially Linda Henley, for supplying some of the questions and for looking over the manuscript;

the Psoriatic Arthropathy Association, especially David Chandler, for their help with supplying questions and looking at the manuscript;

Kath Houson for collecting many questions from patients at the Bristol Royal Infirmary;

the Chandler family for agreeing to be our front cover 'models'.

Any errors are our own.

Foreword

by Professor Andrew Y Finlay

Department of Dermatology, University of Wales College of Medicine, Cardiff

Every year about 20,000 people in the UK develop psoriasis for the first time. Even though so many people are affected, it can be confusing, disturbing and sometimes frightening to be told you have this condition. There are many misunderstandings about this skin disease, and if you have psoriasis you are likely to have lots of questions about it. You need an easy to understand but reliable way to get the answers. This book answers a wide range of real-life questions clearly and accurately.

There is a vast amount of information about psoriasis in the medical literature, as any search on the Internet will quickly reveal. It is, however, very difficult to get this information into perspective, especially if you are not familiar with medical terms. Written by two authors who have great experience of speaking to and helping people with psoriasis in general practice and in a hospital setting, this book can be strongly recommended. For many people with psoriasis it will provide information about everything you want to know.

Psoriasis can affect many different aspects of people's lives – it is not only the coping with treatment that can be difficult but also coping with other people's reactions to the skin changes. The authors clearly understand these concerns, and the questions and answers help to provide advice about many aspects of practical daily coping with psoriasis. They also give positive advice about how to help others understand and accept the condition.

The questions are sensibly divided into sections that deal with different aspects of psoriasis, explaining what it is, what the different types are and what can affect its activity. Treatments are explained and the importance of understanding whether you are taking treatment for which there is proper evidence about effectiveness and safety. Important questions about life-style, relationships and sex, financial matters and how to get the best out of your NHS treatment are answered. The questioners and the authors clearly have their feet on the ground.

This book will be read with interest not only by anyone worried or curious about their own psoriasis but also by their partners, parents and close friends. It will be very useful in helping to clear up misunderstandings and incorrect myths about psoriasis, as well as giving buckets of practical, sensible advice. One day we may have a cure – until then, the information given here will help anyone who has to live with psoriasis.

Andrew Finlay

Introduction

Psoriasis is a recurrent inflammatory skin disease that affects 2–3% of the population in the UK. In simple terms, one person on a full double-decker bus is likely to have the disease. Fair-skinned people, wherever they live, are equally affected by psoriasis, but it is much less common in African Caribbeans and Asians and virtually non-existent in Inuit people and Native Americans. It affects men and women equally. The word 'psoriasis' comes from Greek words meaning 'the state of having the itch', which gives the lie to the suggestion in some medical textbooks that psoriasis does not itch. It also suggests that, although properly described in the 1800s, psoriasis has been around for many centuries.

People's experience of itch can vary from none at all to severe; one in three people say that, for them, itch is the worst aspect of the condition. Life can certainly be made miserable by the itchy, scaly and inflamed 'plaques', which may occur on any part of the skin and scalp. A 'plaque' is the term for the scaly, red, raised patch of skin affected by psoriasis, which can vary in size from 1 to 20 centimetres or more. People may find it disfiguring and it can have a profound effect on their lives. We have some good examples of the misery of the disease in the writings of authors such as John Updike and Dennis Potter, who had a severe form of psoriasis, but we must remember that the severity of the disease is not necessarily linked to its effect on the individual – seemingly trivial psoriasis can cause major psychological problems in some people, whereas others with more severe psoriasis are able to cope better.

Despite the potential impact of psoriasis, many people with this condition do not consult their doctors about it. One estimate indicated that up to 80% of people with the condition did not consult their GP over a period of a year. Reasons for this are probably many and varied, some people disregarding trivial psoriasis and others, with more severe disease, being despondent and fed up with the routine of applying messy creams day in and day out. Some may have had a less than sympathetic response from their GP. One reason for this response might be a lack of training in dermatology, resulting in GPs who are poorly equipped to deal with skin disease even though it can account for 15% of their workload. This omission is being tackled by various bodies such as the Royal College of General Practitioners, the British Association of Dermatologists and Primary Care Dermatology Society groups, representing GPs, consultant dermatologists and GPs with a special interest in dermatology, respectively. Additional support for GP training has come from the All Party Parliamentary Group on Skin and various patient support groups, so it is to be hoped that the recently launched Core Curriculum in Dermatology for GPs in training will make an impact on the care of patients within the next few years.

In the meantime, favourite alternatives to consulting a GP include:

- no treatment at all,
- self-treatment,
- consulting practitioners of complementary therapies,
- holidays around the Dead Sea.

These alternative proposals are very understandable as, even with good quality care, psoriasis can be a very stubborn condition to treat. It also has a remarkable and disheartening tendency to come back even after the skin has been clear for some time.

Many people with psoriasis and the public in general are poorly informed about the disease. Misconceptions abound, causing upset, embarrassment and difficulty in accepting the various treatments. Commonly held beliefs include:

- it's infectious,
- it's an allergy,
- it's to do with the blood,
- it's all caused by stress,
- it will never get better.

None of these is correct. Moreover, psoriasis will get better or worse at times regardless of the treatment being used. It can be difficult to explain why this happens and it is very tempting to look at events preceding such change and see these as the cause. Thus some people might believe that something like a change of diet made them better but this would not apply to anyone else or even to those same people if their psoriasis worsened again. When psoriasis clears completely, either on its own or after treatment, doctors refer to it as being 'in remission' but the length of remission is very variable. This adds to the confusion about what has triggered an attack. What *is* clear is that there are a number of potential trigger factors but the reaction will vary from person to person.

Psoriasis on its own can be a serious disease and more than enough for someone to cope with, but when it is complicated by such things as arthritis it can be very disabling. About 10% of people with psoriasis are thought to have arthritis as well, but the number may be higher. Psoriatic arthropathy (arthritis) is common enough to have its own special name and is a particularly difficult form of arthritis, which may – in one uncommon form – cause severe deformities of the joints in the hands. This can be quite disabling and, when combined with the skin disease, has a major effect on quality of life. Like psoriasis, the arthropathy has been around for thousands of years; the combination of swollen and twisted fingers with scaly skin matches some of the biblical descriptions of lepers, and probably resulted in people with psoriasis being shunned and even isolated from society in leper colonies. This attitude probably continued long after biblical times, as the disease itself wasn't properly described until the nineteenth century. To a certain extent this isolation still occurs today, people with the condition being reluctant to use communal changing facilities, go shopping for clothes or visit a hairdresser for fear of embarrassing stares or even being asked to leave because of others' ignorance about psoriasis.

In today's NHS there is great emphasis on informing and empowering patients, and this applies as much to people with long-term (chronic) skin problems such as psoriasis as to those with other diseases. All patients must have access to simple explanations about their disease, both verbal and in accessible written information sheets. Every contact with a doctor or nurse should allow for questions, however trivial the subject might seem – if it is worth asking, it is worth answering. This book is based on real questions asked by real patients, and we hope that we have provided some useful answers.

We also hope that the book will be read by people without psoriasis as well as those with it, and serve as a way of increasing awareness and understanding of this common disease. Our background is in Western medicine and we do not claim to have all the answers or that our approach is the only valid one, but our aim is to give answers and comments that will provide hope and guidance to many of you.

1
What is psoriasis?

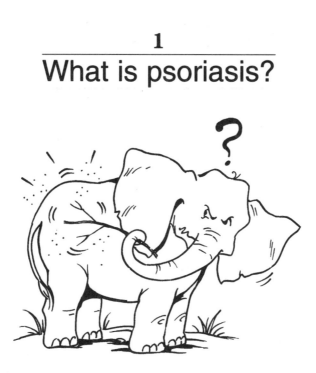

Introduction

Psoriasis is an inflammatory skin condition. The obvious sign is the redness associated with the plaques (the raised patches on the skin), although this is more obvious where there is little scale. Often, however, the white scaling is thick and hides the redness, so, on exposed surfaces, psoriasis looks thick, white and crusty. The thickening is due to the greatly increased 'turnover' of the skin cells. Normally a living skin cell moves upwards from the bottom layer of skin, loses its nucleus and dies. It is then largely made up of a protein called keratin, and is shed from the surface of the skin as new cells go through the same process and replace it from underneath. The whole process takes around 28 days but

5

in psoriasis it is greatly speeded up to a three- to four-day cycle. Living cells are then much closer to the surface and bring their blood supply with them, leading to the redness and heat that many people with psoriasis complain of. Because the surface cells are being replaced before they are shed, this results in a thick layer of scale which, as everyone with the condition knows, flakes off readily and abundantly.

If you gently scratch the surface of a plaque, the scale starts to separate and looks silvery, because it is not as tightly bound down as normal skin. Scratching harder removes the scale, with the appearance of multiple small bleeding points from the increased surface blood supply. Some parts of the body do not have this typical scale. These are usually the areas where two skin surfaces come together (occlusion), as in the natural skin creases and folds (e.g. the groin and genital region and the skin underneath women's breasts). In these areas, psoriasis can look bright red and shiny rather than scaly, because the folds of skin come together, preventing evaporation and increasing the moisture content of the skin. The lesions do not dry out or scale as easily.

The body's immune system plays an important part in this increased cell turnover, as the altered genes in people with psoriasis seem to lead to a change in the function of a skin immune cell type, known as T-lymphocytes or T cells. Lymphocytes make up the bulk of what are called 'white blood cells' and are probably best known for their role in dealing with infection. Their precise role in psoriasis has not been fully worked out but they seem to be able to trigger the increased production of skin cells and attract other cells to the affected skin, which causes the inflammation. The importance of T cells is borne out by the effect that some treatments that alter the function of T cells have on psoriasis. This is discussed in Chapter 5. Because of this subtle way in which the immune system in psoriasis differs from normal, there may be some differences in the tendency for people with psoriasis to be affected by other diseases. Diseases that might be less common include atopic eczema, contact eczema and urticaria (hives). Some skin infections are also less common.

It is equally important to understand what psoriasis is *not*. This can be summarised by saying that it is:

- **not** contagious,
- **not** cancer,
- **not** related to diet, and
- **not** allergic.

A family connection?

My mother and I have psoriasis. Is it hereditary?

Psoriasis can be described as a hereditary disease in that certain genes have been identified as being linked to psoriasis. These genes do not cause psoriasis but they make you more likely to develop it in response to certain 'triggers' that lead to the typical changes in the skin. Medical knowledge of the genes involved is increasing; up to six different genes may be involved, giving rise to the different patterns of psoriasis and different responses to treatment (discussed later in the book). Up to a third of people with the disease have someone in the family who has it as well, and having one particular gene on chromosome 6 (Cw6) makes it 24 times more likely that a person will get psoriasis.

Both my husband and I have psoriasis. Are the chances of our children getting it doubled?

The chances are much more than doubled, presumably due to the chance of inheriting more than one of the 'psoriasis genes'. If only one of you had psoriasis, the chances of your children developing it would be only 15%; because both of you have it, though, the chances rise to 75%.

It is very difficult to answer individual questions about risk: for example, if neither of you had psoriasis but you had a child with the disease, the risk of another child being affected would be 20%.

Are eldest children most likely to get it?

No. All children will have an equal chance of inheriting the gene or genes involved, and there is no evidence to suggest that firstborn children are more likely to be affected by the various factors that can trigger the disease.

I am pregnant and have psoriasis; will my baby have my psoriasis?

Your baby will possibly have an increased risk of developing psoriasis if he or she inherits your 'psoriasis genes', but will not have 'picked it up' from you during the pregnancy even if your psoriasis has been bad. Because genetic material is passed on from both parents when the egg and sperm combine, your baby will only have a 50% chance of getting your genes and therefore a 15% chance of getting psoriasis. This will apply equally to other children you might have.

If my children get psoriasis, will it be as bad as mine?

This is another question that is difficult to answer, because of the interplay between the different genes and trigger factors involved. All we can say, really, is that nobody knows.

I didn't think there was any psoriasis in my family, but my 41-year-old sister has just developed it. What are my chances of getting it, too?

It isn't possible to give you a specific answer, because statistics only work for large groups of people. If you do develop the disease you could look back and say that your risk was 100%, so any answer would be wrong! We hope you don't get it. You may be lucky as, although the overall risk in a case such as yours would be 20%, things are complicated by the age at which your sister developed the disease. Because she developed psoriasis after the age of 30, your risk is three times less than it would be if she had it before the age of 15.

I have twin daughters but only one has psoriasis. Doesn't this suggest that it is not hereditary?

We can understand your confusion. Remember, though, that psoriasis is not caused by the suspect genes; they only make you more *susceptible* to the different triggers. Your daughter without psoriasis is lucky. Studies of large groups of twins help to show the hereditary basis: identical twins have a 65–70% chance of both developing psoriasis but this falls to 15–20% for non-identical twins.

There is psoriasis in my family and I thought I had escaped, but it developed after I was in a bad car accident. Why is this?

This is an example of a trigger factor switching on your inherited tendency to develop psoriasis. Certain things can trigger first or recurrent attacks of psoriasis, or just cause a flare-up of mild disease. These include trauma, infections, hormonal changes, some drugs and other serious illnesses. Good evidence for the importance of trigger factors comes from studying identical twins. Although both have the inherited tendency, there is only a 65–70% chance of both developing psoriasis. Different triggers are important for different people, which is why there can be difficulties in predicting and treating psoriasis.

Why have I contracted the disease when no one else in the family has it?

Although psoriasis is thought to be hereditary, it is really only the *tendency* to get the disease that is passed on in families. Some people can have an abnormal gene capable of causing psoriasis but it is never 'switched on', so the gene could have been passed to you from one of your (unaffected) parents. If not, it would mean that damage to the gene occurred during production of the sperm and egg that you developed from or just after fertilisation. Before you develop psoriasis, some sort of trigger is needed: this could happen at any age, as the disease can appear for the first time in infancy or old age.

Does psoriasis tend to skip a generation?

No. Any pattern in a family suggesting this would have to be explained by looking at trigger factors. It is interesting, though, that there are several other diseases with a reputation for skipping a generation – for example, arthritis and diabetes.

Is it catching?

My husband has psoriasis ever so badly; will I catch it from him?

No. This is a commonly asked question and something that people are understandably concerned about. Psoriasis, like most other skin diseases, is not infectious or catching. People with psoriasis can get very upset by people who avoid touching them because they believe it is contagious, and this can increase the sense of embarrassment and isolation resulting from having different skin. It is very important that you do not 'shy away' from touching your husband, and he might especially value the contact if you help him apply some of his treatments.

Psoriasis and other diseases

Does psoriasis ever turn to skin cancer?

No, there is no evidence that psoriasis is linked to skin cancer. One possible problem, however, arises from the treatment of psoriasis with ultra-violet light, as this can contribute to the kind of skin damage that might turn into cancer if it is not strictly controlled. Many patients also find that their psoriasis improves in the sun, so they may expose themselves more and thus be more at risk of developing a skin cancer. This is explained further in Chapter 5, in the discussion of ultra-violet light treatment.

The scales on my scalp are yellow. Is this another type of psoriasis?

No. You probably have a condition called seborrhoeic eczema in your scalp, which is bad luck if you also have psoriasis elsewhere. Seborrhoeic eczema also causes redness and scaling on the scalp and also on the face and upper body. On the scalp, there are several ways of telling one condition from the other. In seborrhoeic eczema the scales are yellowish and greasy, rather than white and dry. If you pick the scales off, the skin underneath oozes clear fluid and blood all over in seborrhoeic eczema but in psoriasis there are distinct points of bleeding. Seborrhoeic eczema is always itchy but in psoriasis it varies from none to severe.

Can I get eczema as well as psoriasis?

Yes, you can, but it is more likely to be the seborrhoeic form of eczema (mentioned above) than the 'atopic' form, which is the most common type in childhood. There may even be an overlap between seborrhoeic eczema and psoriasis, as it can be difficult to distinguish between the two on the face; some people use the term 'sebopsoriasis'.

How can I tell eczema from psoriasis?

This can be difficult, especially when your hands, feet and scalp are involved. Eczema tends to be more red, wet and weepy with no clear-cut boundary between affected skin and normal skin. Psoriatic 'lesions' are thicker, with a silvery scale and are well demarcated – i.e. it is obvious where the psoriasis stops and normal skin starts. This is equally true for the typical plaques and the bright red patches in flexures (e.g. where the elbow and knee bend) and skin folds where scale is not obvious. As with eczema, psoriasis tends to be symmetrical, which means that it tends to affect both sides of the body (e.g. both knees rather than one or the other). If you have scaly rashes that are not symmetrical, they may be due to some other cause; for example, a fungal infection such as ringworm.

In older people a first appearance of psoriasis tends to be more difficult to diagnose because it can look much more like eczema. Incidentally, their skin is much more likely to be irritated by some of the common treatments.

Is it true that some people with psoriasis are otherwise healthier than other people?

As mentioned in the introduction to this chapter, the importance of the body's immune system in psoriasis means that some conditions may be more or less common in people with psoriasis. Those that may be more common are:

- chronic tonsillitis,
- obesity,
- raised blood pressure,
- heart problems,
- diabetes.

Those that may be less common are:

- atopic eczema,
- allergic asthma,
- urticaria,
- allergic contact eczema.

Over all, though, these differences are not important enough for our answer to your question to be anything other than 'No'.

Miscellaneous

Why is it thought that the immune system plays a part in causing psoriasis?

There are several reasons why the immune system is felt to be important in causing psoriasis. As is discussed in Chapter 5, some immuno-suppressive drugs (which damp down some parts of the body's immune reaction) work well in treating psoriasis. It is also a life-long disease, and this is taken as a sign that there is some 'memory' in the immune system that produces the typical rash of psoriasis in response to certain triggers. This 'memory' is part of the way our immune system works in recognising foreign bacteria and fighting them, and explains why immunisation prevents us developing certain diseases. The way the disease can also clear up without treatment and then flare up again is also typical of a long-term immune response. Finally, some of the genes identified are known to be linked to the way our immune system works.

Once clear, does psoriasis often recur?

Yes. Many patients will testify to this. One person we know has said that the worst thing about having psoriasis is that it 'always comes back'. It is difficult to be specific about individual cases, as, once clear, it can stay away for a long time, but for most people it will recur all too often. About 50% of patients will have a spontaneous remission at some time, with perhaps 10% of them never having another attack.

My plaques feel especially hot. Why is this?

In psoriasis, the normal turnover time for the skin is greatly reduced. Normal skin will be replaced in around 28 days, a slow cycle of new cells forming and turning to flat dead cells as they move up to the surface and are shed. In psoriatic skin this whole process is speeded up to take only a few days. Less mature cells are appearing on the surface of the skin, so the blood vessels that supply them are much closer to the surface than usual. Inflammation is also part of the psoriatic process and this too leads to opening up of the blood vessels. The skin feels hot because of the increased blood flow and, if the psoriasis is very extensive, this can be a serious problem because of the loss of body heat and fluid that evaporates from the hot skin surface. This is explained in Chapter 2.

2

Different types of psoriasis

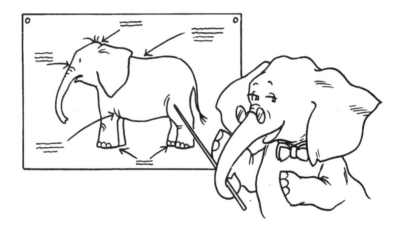

Introduction

As mentioned in Chapter 1, psoriasis is probably determined genetically with an inherited tendency to develop the disease after certain triggers. Up to six different genes may be involved, and this could explain why people can get different patterns of rash. The precise way in which the genes behave has still to be worked out and, as it is possible to inherit more than one of the genes, individual people may have more than one type of the disease, with varying degrees of severity. Until all the genetics are fully worked out, we will have to rely on good descriptions of the patterns of psoriasis to identify the different types, as this can affect the choice of the best treatment approach for each person.

One problem with the many different patterns of psoriasis is that some other conditions may be confused with it. These include eczema in its various forms; *seborrhoeic eczema* (mentioned in Chapter 1) is particularly confusing on the scalp. *Eczema on the hands and feet* can be difficult to tell from psoriasis, and even skin specialists (dermatologists) sometimes have to remove a piece of skin (under local anaesthetic) to be examined under a microscope – called 'doing a biopsy'.

Another confusing pattern is *discoid eczema*. As the name suggests, this occurs in little round areas a few centimetres across, and can be quite thickened. It does not have the typical silvery scaling. Other diseases that may cause confusion are ringworm and a condition called pityriasis rosea. *Ringworm* is more common in children and is usually itchy. It causes round red patches on the body and often on the scalp. These patches can be a bit scaly and tend to grow outwards, leaving a clear area in the middle so they end up looking like a ring. The cause of ringworm is not a worm but a fungus, which also causes athlete's foot. *Pityriasis rosea* is an odd-sounding name but just means 'bran-like' in Greek and 'pink' in Latin! It is a pink rash with fine scaling that appears only round the edge of each lesion, and is thought to be a reaction to a viral infection. It first appears with a single patch 2–5 centimetres across, followed a week or so later by many more smaller oval patches on both sides of the body and upper arms. It can be confused with guttate psoriasis but clears more quickly.

Types of psoriasis

What are the different kinds of psoriasis?

There are many different variations, which may be related to the belief that up to six genes can lead to a person developing psoriasis.

- **Guttate psoriasis** is also known as teardrop or raindrop psoriasis. It tends to occur in children, adolescents and younger adults, and is a generalised rash of small spots up to 1 centimetre in diameter. It tends to follow an infection, often of the throat, when it appears very suddenly a week after the infection. It is widespread but does spare the palms and soles, and clears up after several weeks or months depending on how quickly treatment is started. Up to 50% of people affected will not have a further attack, but it may become chronic or evolve into one of the other types of psoriasis.

- **Plaque psoriasis** is the 'typical' form with scaly, red, raised patches – the plaques – which vary in size from a few millimetres to many centimetres. They tend to be symmetrical and prefer the 'extensor' surfaces such as the backs of the elbows and the fronts of the knees. The lower back and sacral area (top of the buttocks) is another common site for large plaques. Although the plaques can be very large and widespread, they generally cover 5% or less of a person's body surface.

- **Flexural psoriasis** occurs in skin folds, armpits, under the breasts, in the groins and between the buttocks. It is described separately because the appearance is much less scaly, often being quite a bright shiny red colour. In the groins it can also affect the genitals. It can cause troublesome nappy rash in infants but is mainly found in older people. The reason for the lack of scale is the decreased water loss from two surfaces of skin lying against each other.

- **Scalp psoriasis** is often very troublesome, with thick scale and redness that is also evident around the scalp margins. Nevertheless, the hair growth is not usually affected. Even if more hair falls out than normal, it all grows back again.

- **Psoriasis on the face** is relatively uncommon and can be less clearly demarcated, leading to confusion with eczema.

- **Pustular psoriasis** can affect just the hands and feet, with round yellow pustules (raised areas of skin containing pus) appearing under the skin surface of the palms or soles, or both. They gradually turn brown as they reach the surface and are shed as scales. The pustules are sterile and not due to infection. This pattern is most often seen in middle-aged people who are smokers. *Generalised pustular psoriasis*, with sheets of very small pustules on a background of very red, hot skin, is a medical emergency. A person can become very ill from loss of heat and fluid, and feel very feverish. It is sometimes triggered if large amounts of strong steroid creams have been used to treat widespread plaques or after oral steroids.

- **Erythrodermic psoriasis** also is an emergency. Like many medical terms, erythroderma is from the Greek – for 'red' or 'inflamed' and 'skin'. The whole of the skin turns red and leads to loss of fluid and heat, as with pustular psoriasis. There are no pustules but urgent admission to hospital is needed to replace lost fluid and to prevent hypothermia (low body temperature). The underlying psoriasis also needs to be treated once the person has been stabilised. Erythroderma can occur with other skin diseases such as eczema but is, thankfully, quite rare. It can occur slowly but, as with pustular psoriasis, often develops suddenly after incorrect use or sudden withdrawal of steroid treatment.

- **Psoriasis of the nails**. There can often be changes to the nails. These range from discoloration and pitting of the surface to complete destruction of the nail because the psoriasis can make the nails split away from the nail bed and cause considerable thickening of the skin from under the nail. Severe nail changes can be very disabling and should never be dismissed as just being a 'cosmetic' problem.

- **Psoriatic arthropathy**. A final and very distressing type of psoriasis is that with arthritis. Psoriatic arthropathy may occur in up to 10% of people with psoriasis; it has a pattern similar to that of rheumatoid arthritis, with the possibility of serious deformity. The true number of people with this type of arthritis is very difficult to judge, as there is a lot of overlap with other types of arthritis. Of people with severe psoriasis, some 21% might be affected with arthritis of varying severity.

What is gutter psoriasis?

I think you mean guttate psoriasis. Guttate means 'drop-like' and is used to describe a type of psoriasis that is often the first manifestation in adolescents and young adults. It is an example of infection triggering the disease and often follows a sore throat, especially when a bacterium called *Streptococcus* is the cause. Very small drop-like patches of psoriasis appear on the trunk and limbs, and may slowly clear on their own after several months. This can look quite dramatic, sometimes like having been splattered with red paint. Having an attack of guttate psoriasis does not necessarily mean that you will go on to develop other forms of the disease, but it may return if you suffer from the same type of sore throat again.

Is there any way of preventing nails from pitting?

No. Pitting occurs when psoriasis affects the nail as it is formed. The tough horny layer forming the nail is weakened and partially collapses, forming the pits 1 millimetre or less in diameter. They are usually scattered randomly on the nail, and can affect finger and toe nails.

I have psoriasis in my ears. Will I go deaf?

The ear canals leading from the outside to the eardrum are simply rolled-up tubes of skin, so psoriasis can occur there. It will not cause permanent deafness from damage to your ears, but can lead to the canal being blocked with scales and wax, muffling your hearing. Treatment can be difficult and you might need to have your ears cleaned out at the ear, nose and throat (ENT) department of your local hospital. Quite often, though, this can be treated successfully with eardrops prescribed by your doctor. Do not be tempted to try to clean out your ears with cotton buds, as this can compact the debris at the end of the canal and make the problem far worse.

Can I get it in my mouth?

It is possible to get psoriasis in the mouth, as it can affect mucous membranes – the term for the lining of internal surfaces such as the mouth and gut. This is quite rare, though, and tends to occur only with severe psoriasis, especially the pustular type (explained in the *Introduction* to this chapter). There is a weak link between psoriasis and a condition called 'geographic tongue' in which the surface of the tongue varies in texture and colour from loss of the normal roughness and increased reddening of the smoother areas. It can look like the outline on a map, hence the name.

Psoriatic arthropathy

What is psoriatic arthropathy?

As if it were not enough to have psoriasis, some people have the added problem of a form of arthritis specific to psoriasis – psoriatic arthropathy. This is probably more common than the quoted 10% of people with the skin disease, because mild cases are often not reported and there is also overlap with other forms of arthritis. Psoriatic arthropathy might also go unreported because of the different patterns of arthritis, which might not always be recognised as being linked to psoriasis and the fact that it can appear before the skin is affected.

The arthritis appears with pain and tenderness over one or more joints. In the larger joints and the spine this pain can be quite intense. If the smaller joints of the hands and feet are affected, there can be a lot of stiffness in the mornings or after periods of rest or inactivity.

Five patterns of psoriatic arthropathy are distinct enough to be mentioned separately. As with all classifications, though, they are very general and someone might have features of more than one type.

- The most common pattern accounts for just over half the cases and affects the end joints of the fingers and toes. It usually occurs on only one side of the body (asymmetrical), and tends to affect the fingers or toes where there are nail changes as well.
- About a quarter of cases have symmetrical arthritis (on both sides of the body), which resembles rheumatoid arthritis but does not give a positive result to the blood test for rheumatoid factor, which is in the bloodstream of people with rheumatoid

arthritis. It affects many joints at the same time, and can be found in both small joints and larger ones such as the hips and knees. This can be a very troublesome form of the disease, as about half the people who have it get worse with slow destruction of the joints.

- The next most common pattern is where the arthritis affects the spine; pain and stiffness are felt in the lower back and parts of the body where large muscles are attached to bones via the tendons. This causes problems around the Achilles tendon (at the ankle) and the pelvis (the hip).
- Least common is the pattern that affects just large joints and on only one side of the body.
- Lastly, there is a very destructive form of the disease, called arthritis mutilans. As the name suggests, it is a severe, deforming arthritis that affects the small joints of the hands and also the feet and spine.

With psoriatic arthritis, does the psoriasis rash on the skin appear at the same time as the arthritis?

Usually the skin rash comes first, but in a few cases the arthritis appears first and it can be many years before psoriasis is seen on the skin. Occasionally, everything develops together. If you have an odd pattern of arthritis and no skin problems, your doctor might look very closely at your nails in case they show the pitting typical of psoriatic nail changes. You might also want to ask your relatives if anyone in the family is known to have psoriasis, as this could make it more likely that your joint problems are linked to it.

My fingers have swollen up. I've read that you can have arthritis with psoriasis. Could this be my problem?

You could have one of the types of arthritis linked with psoriasis. It depends on where the swelling appears. If it affects just the last joint of your fingers, perhaps where you have some nail changes, and is not the same on both hands, it is likely to be due to the most common form of arthritis associated with psoriasis. This is unlikely to get much worse and will not affect the rest of your joints.

If, however, other finger joints and/or your knuckles are affected and it is the same on both hands, you have a more progressive form of the disease. If this is the case, you should see your doctor as soon as possible.

The swelling of arthritis is usually accompanied by pain, tenderness and stiffness. If you don't have any of these other problems, you might have swelling from another cause, such as infection or fluid retention, which need completely different treatment.

Is there a blood test I can have for the arthritis associated with my psoriasis?

No, there isn't. It would be much simpler if there were a test but this type of arthritis is called 'sero-negative' because nothing shows up when the serum part of the blood is tested. It is important, though, to do this test if the arthritis is symmetrical, as it can be confused with rheumatoid arthritis, which is 'sero-positive' – more than 80% of people with this disease have a substance called rheumatoid factor in their blood.

A test you might be offered looks at levels of inflammation in your body, and can be useful in deciding if your arthritis is very active or not. It can look at the 'ESR' (erythrocyte sedimentation rate – the speed at which red blood cells settle under gravity) or 'viscosity' (stickiness of your blood), which would be raised if you had a lot of inflammation.

These tests are not helpful in deciding whether you have psoriatic arthropathy, because they indicate inflammation from any cause, such as severe infection or some diseases that cause inflammation in the gut.

Is it possible for me to have arthritis that is not caused by my psoriasis?

Yes, indeed. Just because you have psoriasis it does not mean that any aches and pains should be labelled as being due to psoriatic arthropathy. You are just as likely as people without psoriasis to have osteo- or rheumatoid arthritis, or even conditions such as gout that can be confused with the type of psoriatic arthritis that affects only one joint. Only 4% of people with generalised arthritis have the psoriatic form. Although the early treatment of painful joints may be much the same regardless of the cause, it is important for you to discuss things with your GP and make sure you are having any appropriate tests. There are developments in imaging techniques using MRI (magnetic resonance imaging) scanners that might make it easy to diagnose psoriatic arthropathy in the future.

I have only a little bit of psoriasis but have some painful joints. Isn't it just people with lots of psoriasis who get the arthritis?

No, unfortunately anyone with psoriasis can get joint problems – sometimes before they know they have a skin disease. People with severe psoriasis are, however, more likely than others to get arthritis, because they have almost a one in four chance compared with a one in ten chance over all.

Cause or effect?

Sometimes I pick off the top layer of scaly plaque. Does this damage my skin in any way?

It will not lead to permanent direct damage, but can cause problems because the skin will bleed very easily under the scale and you could introduce infection. Plaques tend to get very itchy as they dry out and many patients do scratch or, like you, try to pick off the scales to stop the itch. It would be much better to rub in a moisturising cream.

How can I stop the irritation?

The best way to stop the irritation is, of course, to treat the psoriasis so that it clears up. This is often easier said than done, but simply moisturising the skin with a greasy preparation can help greatly. It will also prevent the plaques from drying out and cracking, which can make them very sore – a common problem in cold dry weather.

I recently had my appendix out and now have psoriasis in the scar. Why is this?

This is an example of a very common and troublesome problem for people with psoriasis. The disease can occur after any damage to the skin such as a wound or even a bad scratch. This is called Koebner's phenomenon after a German dermatologist who described the reaction in the nineteenth century. It also occurs with other skin problems such as warts.

When the psoriasis falls from my scalp, is it 'dead skin'? I have found that when a piece falls onto a part of my body it irritates, makes me scratch and a patch appears later. Am I imagining this or is the psoriasis still alive?

The scale falling from your scalp is dead and cannot cause psoriasis anywhere else. Even a living cell picked out from a patch of psoriasis would not affect any other part of your skin, because psoriasis is not infectious and cannot be 'caught'. The scale falling on your skin creates a sensation that you may interpret as itch. It could be that the resulting scratching gives rise to a patch of psoriasis in your skin, as it already has the potential to develop the disease. This is another example of the 'Koebner phenomenon' mentioned above.

Wherever I go, I leave a snowstorm of scales behind me – how can I reduce this?

This is a common and difficult problem for people with psoriasis, who sometimes find it restrictive and embarrassing. Leaving snowstorms can make it very difficult to stay in other people's homes and to do everyday things such as wearing dark clothes or trying on clothes. As with irritation, though, it can be helped by using a moisturiser frequently throughout the day. Some people notice that their psoriasis dries up and sheds more scale as it starts to get better, so welcome this as a good sign.

3

What triggers psoriasis and what makes it worse?

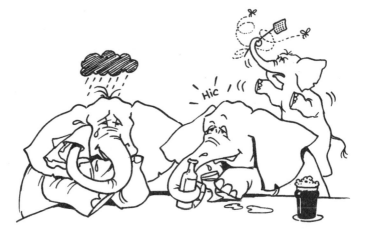

Introduction

As mentioned earlier in this book, genetic changes can give you the tendency to develop psoriasis but some trigger is needed to start the process off. A variety of trigger factors have been identified but more research is needed, especially into why some areas of the skin will develop psoriatic plaques whereas other areas remain normal. It can be very difficult to make generalisations from what we call 'anecdotal evidence' of individual patients' reports about triggers but the list below reflects the events or things that do seem able to have an effect on people with psoriasis at some time.

- Stress and emotional upset.
- Infection.
- Injury to the skin – even a simple scratch or insect bite.
- Puberty, menopause and pregnancy.
- Some prescribed drugs (e.g. beta-blockers, chloroquine, lithium).
- Alcohol in excess.
- Smoking.
- Poor general health.
- Changes in climate.
- Severe damage to the immune system (e.g. with AIDS, or after chemotherapy for cancer).
- Exposure to ultra-violet light (rarely).

Diet

Does diet affect psoriasis?

There is little scientific evidence that suggests a direct link between diet and psoriasis. It is wise for everyone to have a healthy balanced diet that contains lots of fresh fruit and vegetables (at least five portions per day) and to drink plenty of fluids (1.5–2 litres), especially water. Following these sensible guidelines will help you to stay healthy, which will have a beneficial effect on your skin. It is worth saying that some people believe very strongly that certain foods do make their skin feel worse. If you think this is the case and you can identify foods that worsen your skin, it is worth avoiding or reducing them.

It may be that you have an additional problem called urticaria (or hives), which can be triggered by certain foods, and you should discuss this further with your GP. Urticaria is not related to psoriasis and is not caused by a reaction to food.

When I drink a lot of alcohol, my skin feels worse the next day. Why is this?

Alcohol has the effect of dehydrating the body (i.e. removing excessive amounts of water), which is one reason why a headache is part of a hangover. This dehydration also affects the skin and causes it to become drier. Consequently, if you have had excessive amounts of alcohol, you are likely to make your psoriasis drier – which will make it feel worse. Having one or two alcoholic drinks in an evening should not have an adverse effect, but drinking enough to get drunk or having more than 10 units in one evening may make your skin worse.

Sometimes people find themselves drinking excessive alcohol as a way of coping with their psoriasis. This is not a helpful coping strategy and, as highlighted here, will actually make your skin worse. Some of the treatments for severe psoriasis (e.g. methotrexate – discussed in Chapter 5) make it dangerous to drink alcohol. Methotrexate is broken down in the liver, as is alcohol. Drinking alcohol when taking methotrexate can put an extra strain on the liver, which may damage it.

There is some evidence that alcohol can be involved in triggering psoriasis – a suggestion that is denied by many people. We have been told by some patients that if we had psoriasis, we would drink too!

Stress

Is psoriasis affected by rest or stress?

The role that stress plays in psoriasis is somewhat controversial. It is helpful to consider two extreme points of view. For some people there is a very clear relation between stressful events and psoriasis flaring up. This connection is so direct that they can feel the psoriasis getting worse or throbbing when they are in a difficult situation. Other people cannot find any direct relation between experiencing stressful events and their psoriasis flaring up. The simple answer, then, is that stress can make psoriasis worse, and for most people the role that stress plays is somewhere between the two examples given here.

Sometimes it is difficult to identify the stressful event that has made the psoriasis worse; it may be that a period of time passes between a stressful event and the psoriasis getting worse. The other issue that is very clear is that having psoriasis itself is a stress. Thus getting a flare-up of psoriasis may set off a vicious circle whereby the flare-up causes stress, which makes the psoriasis worse, which causes stress . . . Effective and timely treatments are of particular importance, as they help to break the vicious circle or even stop it from starting in the first place.

Rest is important, and finding time to unwind from a busy work or home life helps to keep stress under control. Simple things such as having enough sleep help to increase your resilience and to decrease the effect of a stressful life-style. A rest from the seemingly endless routine of applying creams to your skin can also help greatly. This can be achieved by letting trained nurses apply the creams in the out-patient clinic or even during a short spell in hospital as an in-patient.

If psoriasis is stress related, what can be done to reduce levels of stress?

This is a difficult question to answer, because everyone is different in terms of what helps them to reduce stress.

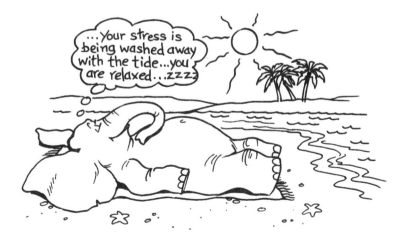

However, there are a number of strategies that it is useful to consider.

First of all, you can identify the factors that cause you most stress in your life and consider whether it is possible to change or avoid them. It may be useful to sit down and talk about these with someone close to you or your own nurse/doctor. It is sometimes difficult to do this alone because you are so close to the stress factors that it is hard to recognise them. If you cannot remove or change the things that cause you stress (e.g. it may not be possible to change your job or get rid of your kids!), you need to use strategies that help you relax and create time for yourself. This is where individual preference comes in. For some people, playing sport might provide a therapeutic outlet for stress. For others, having a massage, trying reflexology or starting meditation may provide the answers. The underlying message of this advice is to create space and time for yourself to allow you to do something that makes you feel good. The temptation may be to indulge in something that makes you feel good in the short term but has no real long-term benefits (e.g. heavy drinking). This sort of destructive activity is known as a negative coping strategy and, rather than helping the situation, will probably make it worse.

The second thing that can be done to reduce stress levels is to get effective treatment. Psoriasis and stress tend to be a vicious circle – stress can trigger psoriasis which, when it appears, makes you feel more stressed, which makes your psoriasis worse, and so on. Getting treatment that makes your skin feel and look better and that fits in with your life-style can break the vicious circle.

To summarise, you need a two-pronged plan to remedy the impact of stress. First, a mental approach that helps you to relax more and create time for yourself and, secondly, a physical approach to ensure that your psoriasis has a minimal physical impact.

Other triggers of flare-ups

What usually makes psoriasis flare up?

As mentioned in the answer above, stressful life-styles and specific stressful events are thought to be a possible cause or 'trigger' of flare-ups.

Certain drugs are also known to aggravate psoriasis – these include the anti-malarial drug chloroquine, the anti-depressant lithium, and anti-arrhythmic drugs and beta-blockers usually used to treat heart disease. It may be that if you are taking any of these drugs you cannot discontinue them, and you certainly should not do so without consulting your doctor. However, it is worth discussing it with your doctor, as there may be alternatives that do not have a triggering effect.

A throat infection – especially 'strep' (caused by *Streptococcus* bacteria) – can trigger guttate psoriasis. (See also the next question and Chapters 1 and 2 for further details.)

Damaging the skin (e.g. a cut from falling over or from surgery) can trigger psoriasis at the point of the injury. This is known as Koebner's phenomenon (named after the man who first described it). The skin does not have to be broken for this to occur. Many of you will be familiar with the fact that psoriasis develops where your clothes rub (e.g. round the belt line); this too is Koebner's phenomenon, caused by the constant rubbing of material against the skin. Scratching itchy patches of psoriasis may also aggravate the psoriasis because scratching can damage the skin.

For most people sunshine is very helpful in improving the psoriasis, but for about 10% of people with psoriasis sunlight actually makes the condition worse.

My doctor says I have got it because of a sore throat.

Guttate psoriasis, a specific type of psoriasis in which a lot of small raindrop-like spots appear across the body, is often triggered by a streptococcal throat infection. It is this infection that gives you the sore throat. Your doctor may advise you to see him or her whenever you have a sore throat, so that you can be treated with antibiotics. This may stop the psoriasis from developing.

Can an infection cause psoriasis to flare up?

As mentioned in the previous answer, a streptococcal infection can lead to a flare-up of guttate psoriasis. Other sorts of infections may aggravate psoriasis in that they make you feel generally more run down and thus more susceptible to the stresses of everyday life. However, there is not the same direct connection that there is between the streptococcal infection and guttate psoriasis.

My psoriasis always better in the winter than in the summer, but my cousin's is better in the summer. Why is this?

It is fair to say that your cousin's situation is more usual than your own. Most people find that, as soon as they are able to expose their skin to the sunshine in summer, their psoriasis shows some signs of improvement. For many people the cold, dark winter months make their skin worse. It may be that you are one of the few people (about 10%) for whom sunshine makes the skin worse, which is why your skin is better in winter than summer.

Does biological washing powder make it worse?

Unlike eczema, psoriasis does not tend to be sensitive to external 'sensitisers' – irritants that cause the skin to become inflamed. So the simple answer is that it is very unlikely. However, if you were sensitive to washing powder anyway or had an irritant reaction to an ingredient that meant your skin was damaged (either through the rash or through you scratching), psoriasis might develop because of Koebner's phenomenon (see earlier in this chapter).

Is psoriasis linked to fungal changes?

Having a fungal infection – athlete's foot or ringworm – does not cause psoriasis but some types of fungus may infect nails damaged by the disease. Some of the nail changes in psoriasis and fungal infection can look very similar, so it is worth checking this out – especially if only a few nails are affected. Your GP should be able to arrange for nail clippings to be examined for evidence of fungal infection. Some fungal infections can look very like small patches of psoriasis with redness and scale.

Is psoriasis linked to hormonal fluctuations?

Some women report that their psoriasis seems to vary according to their monthly cycle but there is no clear scientific evidence for this. Likewise, most women find that during pregnancy their psoriasis improves, only to return once they have given birth. However, the reverse is also true, as other women find that their psoriasis gets worse during pregnancy. In women, psoriasis often starts at puberty or the menopause, which does suggest that the changes in hormone levels may trigger psoriasis.

It might seem logical to think that, if hormonal changes apparently trigger psoriasis, a possible treatment would be hormone therapy. Unfortunately, the link between the hormonal changes and developing psoriasis are not that straightforward, and hormone treatment is not being seriously investigated at present.

4
First-line treatments

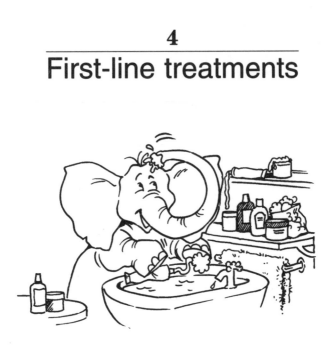

Introduction

Because psoriasis can come and go over a lifetime, it is
important that people with the disease feel empowered to
manage it themselves. Health care professionals should provide
help, education, support and treatment advice when necessary.
Treating psoriasis should be a team effort, the team members
varying according to the needs of the person concerned.
Treatments need to be acceptable to the individual as well as
being effective, so it is important that health care professionals
understand your view of the disease. The cost of treatment in
both time and money has to be taken into account, and the
chore of applying creams once or twice a day can dampen one's

motivation to treat the skin over a prolonged period. So it is very important to avoid looking at the psoriasis on its own, because treatment is much more likely to succeed if it is firmly grounded in the context of your life, beliefs and needs for treatment. Expectations, especially unrealistic ones, must be explored and discussed.

'First-line treatments' are the initial treatments that the doctor or nurse will suggest to manage your psoriasis. For mild to moderate psoriasis they are usually all that are required to control it successfully. If the psoriasis is severe and/or doesn't respond to first-line treatments, the doctor may recommend a move on to second-line treatments (discussed in the next chapter).

First-line treatments generally involve applying creams and ointments to the skin (topical treatment); when used properly, they have minimal side (unwanted) effects. There are lots of different treatments on the market, often with a bewildering variety of names, and many manufacturers make extravagant claims about their success. However, the fundamental components of first-line treatments usually belong to a fairly limited list.

Whatever treatment you use, *moisturisers will be the mainstay.*

Emollients are substances used to moisturise the skin either by being rubbed in or by putting them in the bath or shower. There is a huge range available and every individual should be able to find an acceptable one. More descriptions and explanations for the use of emollients are given in this chapter.

Tar is a useful substance to treat psoriasis although it tends to have a strong smell and can be very messy. Tar-based products range from weak substances (e.g. in Alphosyl) to much stronger ones (e.g. coal tar and salicylic acid ointment, which tends to be prepared and used in hospital departments). Although there is no conclusive evidence linking the use of coal tar with cancer, there have been concerns about a risk in people who use it extensively over long periods of time. Tar can be used on small or large plaques of psoriasis; although it can irritate unaffected skin, this is only temporary and mild, and makes tar suitable for psoriasis plaques that do not have a definite edge and/or are widespread across the body. It is not generally recommended for delicate areas of skin (e.g. skin folds or the face), but can be very useful for pustular psoriasis on the hands and feet.

Dithranol, now manufactured chemically, was originally extracted from a special tree bark extract. Its value in psoriasis was discovered by accident when a patient with psoriasis and arthritis was given a powder produced from the tree to treat the arthritis. His psoriasis cleared even though the arthritis did not. Dithranol is now used to treat well-defined plaques of psoriasis. It can irritate quite seriously if it is allowed to get onto skin with no psoriasis on it, so it needs to be applied carefully. It is usually applied for only a short period of time before being washed off. It doesn't smell but it does tend to stain clothes and surrounding furniture a distinctive purple colour.

Vitamin D derivatives – for example, Dovonex (calcipotriol) and Curatoderm (tacalcitol) – are newer treatments for psoriasis, and have the advantage of being relatively clean and non-smelly. They are easy to apply, and, although some irritation has been experienced by some people, this is usually fairly mild and only temporary.

Vitamin A derivatives – for example, Zorac (tazarotene) – are the newest topical treatment for psoriasis. They are applied once a day and can be used for up to 12 weeks. The face and skin folds should be avoided because it can cause irritation. The preparations are relatively clean and non-smelly.

Topical steroids are not used routinely for treating chronic plaque psoriasis because, although potent or very potent steroids can have a very spectacular positive effect, the psoriasis often comes back (rebounds) as bad if not worse than before once they have been stopped. However, short-term use of steroids can be very helpful, especially when psoriasis is inflamed or when it exists in delicate areas of the skin (e.g. skin folds or the face).

Topical treatments often take four to eight weeks to have any effect, which can be quite demoralising. However, they can work very well and the best strategy is to choose treatments that fit best into your life-style. It is very important that you use the correct amount of cream or ointment: some treatments need to be applied sparingly whereas others are put on more thickly. Many people notice that, if one or two plaques start to fade with the treatment, the others do so of their own accord. If treating all the psoriasis seems too much trouble, it is worth tackling the bits that are most bothersome and seeing if the others fade by themselves. We would always recommend that you put moisturiser on all over the body, as this really does help to soothe and smooth.

What sort of treatment?

How does my doctor decide which treatment is most suitable for me?

Your doctor will make the decisions about what treatments are most suitable for you based on two main factors.

- The extent and location of your psoriasis will be a major consideration. Some treatments are suitable for mild to moderate psoriasis but would not be as helpful for severe psoriasis. Similarly, some treatments are suitable for your trunk, arms and legs but not for your face.
- Your life-style will also influence what your doctor prescribes. He or she should check with you such issues as how much time you have to give to doing treatments, whether you have a partner who can help you and what sort of job you do. These are all important, because, whatever treatment you are prescribed, you have to be willing and able to use it – treatments do not help psoriasis if they stay in their pots!

When I apply the creams to treat my psoriasis, what should I expect to see by way of improvement?

There are a number of changes that you should see if you are using the treatments properly and often enough. Applying moisturisers regularly will make your plaques less scaly and less itchy, softer and more flexible; however, this is unlikely to make the plaques themselves smaller. Whichever type of 'active' treatment you are using (e.g. tar, dithranol or vitamin D creams), you will notice that the psoriasis tends to fade from the centre of the plaque outwards. The plaques themselves will not shrink in size but clear areas of skin will appear in the centre of the plaque, leaving outer rings that will be the last to clear. You can also tell by touch that the centre is clear by running your finger over it and feeling how smooth it is. Dithranol, uniquely, temporarily stains the skin a purple/brown colour. This staining occurs only on skin cleared of psoriasis, so you know when the psoriasis has gone because your skin starts to stain! The stain will disappear within a couple of weeks.

How long does it take for the plaques to disappear when I use the creams?

The length of time that it takes to clear the psoriasis varies from person to person. If the plaques are very thick to begin with, it will take longer to clear them than if they are thin and not scaly. It also depends on which treatments you are using and how effectively you are applying them. Having said this, as a general rule you should reckon on four to eight weeks of regular treatment (according to the instructions) before clearance occurs, although there will be improvement before this. Because it takes this length of time, it is especially important that you find a treatment that fits into your life-style and that is as easy as possible to use.

Does treatment need to be ongoing?

Once your skin is clear of psoriasis, you need only continue to use moisturisers (lotions are often sufficient). However, keep your eyes open for any new spots appearing, as it is easier to treat these when they are new and small rather than waiting until they get bigger.

What is the success rate of available treatments?

Most treatments mentioned in this chapter have a good success rate when used properly (regularly and in conjunction with moisturisers). The difficulty that most people experience is trying to keep up regular treatments – i.e. fitting twice-daily regimens into everyday life. You may in the end decide that you are content to keep your psoriasis comfortable and under control and that complete clearance is unrealistic because the treatment regimens just do not fit into your life-style. This point of view is absolutely fine as long as you are happy with it.

Does perspiration help to clear up psoriasis?

No, it doesn't. In fact, some people find that getting hot and sweating aggravates the symptoms of their psoriasis.

Are there any restrictions to my treatments?

It is difficult to answer this question without knowing your exact treatments, but the following points can be made to establish some general principles. First, moisturising is a key component of treatment and you can never use too much moisturiser. Most of the other treatments do have recommended amounts for usage as well as length of time over which they should be used. For example:

- **Steroids**   These should be used with caution and only over a short period of time. They are rarely used on their own for chronic plaque psoriasis because, although they make it better initially, when they are stopped the psoriasis can come back worse than before. They are, however, useful for inflamed psoriasis, psoriasis in flexures (groins, underarms and under breasts) and on the face. In each box of steroid there is a guidance sheet for the correct amount to use measured in 'fingertip units'.
- **Vitamin D derivatives**   The recommended quantity for these is not more than 100g over a period of a week in an adult. Over-use can interfere with the body's absorption of calcium.
- **Coal tar/Dithrocream**   There is no real restriction to the amount of these that you can use, but over-use can make your skin sore and uncomfortable. They are not recommended for use on the more delicate parts of your skin – i.e. your face and in your flexures.

Moisturisers

Why should I use moisturisers?

Although there is little scientific research into the effects of moisturisers on psoriasis, our own experience shows that:

- moisturisers make the skin *much* more comforable – they decrease the dryness, scaling, cracking and soreness, and itching;
- moisturisers allow the other active treatments you use (e.g. tar, vitamin D) to work more effectively.

Which moisturiser is best to use?

There are so many to choose from that sometimes it is difficult to know. There are, however, two golden rules:

- Moisturising is absolutely vital for anyone with psoriasis. Although it does not get rid of the psoriasis, it makes it less scaly and much more comfortable.
- The best moisturiser is the one that you feel happiest with and that you feel you can use easily on a regular basis. Discuss this with your GP and ask her or him to prescribe one that you like and will use.

Below are some other things to think about when you are choosing a moisturiser.

CONSISTENCY

Lotions are water based and tend to be very runny and easy to apply. They are quite cooling but not very good at moisturising particularly dry skin. They are useful for maintaining good skin once the psoriasis goes (e.g. E45 lotion).

Creams are thicker and a bit greasier than lotions but are still easy to use. They are less runny and tend to come in pots or pump dispensers. They are usually the best option for day-to-day use (e.g. Diprobase).

Ointments are very greasy and thick, and are oil rather than water based. They are the best moisturisers but are less pleasant to use because they are greasy and quite sticky. However, if your skin is very dry, they are the best option (e.g. Epaderm or 50/50 white soft paraffin/liquid paraffin mix).

FREQUENCY

You should use your moisturiser at least twice a day and more often if possible. Try to make your treatment fit in with your life-style as best you can. Some suggestions might be to use a lighter cream moisturiser in the morning before going to work or school and then using a greasier ointment before going to bed. Try taking a small pot of cream to work with you and applying it if a patch gets particularly dry, itchy or uncomfortable. If you are applying a moisturiser all over, it is very easy to get through a 500g pot in a month, so make sure your doctor prescribes enough.

METHOD OF APPLICATION

When you apply the moisturiser you should do this by gently stroking the cream/ointment on in a way that follows the line of your hair. Try not to rub too aggressively, as this will only serve to aggravate the plaques – a gentle repeated motion is best.

IN THE BATH OR SHOWER

Moisturising is not just about putting cream or ointments on; it starts in the bath or shower. As indicated in the answer to a question later, in the section *Practical aspects*, it is wise to wash with a soap substitute that does not dry your skin. If you choose to bath, put a bath oil in the water; this helps to create a layer of oil over the skin, which prevents moisture from being lost from the skin. Beware the risk of slipping when you get in and out of the bath or shower!

To summarise, moisturising should involve:

- using a soap substitute,
- putting an oil in the bath (e.g. Balneum or Oilatum),
- using lots of cream or ointment moisturisers at least twice a day,
- choosing the moisturisers that suit you and your life-style best.

When should I apply moisturisers?

As mentioned in the answer above, moisturisers should be applied as often as possible. However, there are two key times when moisturisers are a must:

- Straight after a bath or shower, because the skin is warm and absorbs the moisturiser better.
- Before putting on a treatment. It is important that the moisturiser is absorbed into the skin, because if it is sitting on the surface of your skin it may make the active treatment less effective.

A good routine to get into is to bath or shower using a soap substitute, apply moisturiser and allow it to sink into the skin and then apply the active treatment. (This is virtually instant if you are using a lotion, takes 10–15 minutes with a cream but may take 45 minutes to an hour with an ointment.) You should repeat the process at either end of the day although clearly you only need to bath or shower once. Any other moisturiser that you can apply through out the day is a bonus.

I keep hearing people talking about emollient therapy. What is this, and is there a difference between this and moisturisers?

The only difference between emollients and moisturisers is the words, rather than their meaning; they mean essentially the same thing. However, sometimes the phrase 'emollient therapy' is used to refer to the whole procedure described in the answer to an earlier question – i.e. the use of soap substitutes and bath oil as well as applying the creams or ointments. In this context, 'moisturisers' usually refer to the creams and ointments themselves.

What is the difference between creams and ointments? I thought all the things you put on your skin were creams.

Although there is a difference between creams and ointments, it can get a bit confusing because people refer to all the substances that go on the skin as creams. Strictly speaking, creams are water based, tend to be white in colour and are quickly absorbed into the skin. Although they are good moisturisers, they are not as effective as ointments, which are oil based. They tend to be translucent (although not always) and are very good moisturisers. So moisturisers can be either a cream or an ointment.

But to make life more complicated, other treatments can come in cream or ointment form. For example, most steroid applications come in either an ointment or a cream, as do vitamin D applications. As mentioned in an earlier answer, although ointments have a better moisturising effect they tend to be less pleasant to use. It is personal preference and you need to decide for yourself which preparations you like best. GPs often prescribe the ointment form of vitamin D and steroid treatments. If you find these too 'tacky' or sticky, ask your GP to prescribe you the cream form.

My doctor has given me Dovonex. Should I still be using moisturisers?

Yes! Yes! Yes! No matter what other treatment your doctor gives you, you should always use moisturiser before applying the other treatment. Once it has sunk in, the moisturiser makes the other treatments – such as calcipotriol (e.g. Dovonex) – more effective, as well as easier to apply, by reducing the scale and allowing better absorption of the active creams.

Coal tar

Coal tar was the best for me. Why can't I still get it?

Many chemists have stopped making up coal tar solutions in white soft paraffin. This is because legislation has meant that they need more safety equipment to manufacture coal tar preparations and most chemists do not have these facilities. The treatments are still available in hospital dermatology departments but rarely in high street chemist shops. Clearly, weak tar-based products such as Alphosyl and Cocois are still available.

I have read a lot about Exorex and understand that it is now available on prescription. Is it worth trying?

Exorex is the brand name for a group of treatments for psoriasis. There is a *lotion* that is a weak tar solution (and has the characteristic tar smell), and also a *moisturiser* and a *shampoo* (these do not contain tar). Tar is a useful treatment for psoriasis and is helpful for many people. The amount of tar in Exorex is low but the lotion is easy to put on. The moisturiser contains an extract from the banana plant, which is what has received a lot of media attention. It is a cream and is slightly greasy (see Appendix 2). It is really a matter of personal preference as to whether you like it more than any of the other emollients.

Steroids

My cousin's doctor has suggested that he might need to use steroids for his psoriasis. What do steroids actually do?

Steroids are essentially hormones and there are many different types with quite different actions. The human body makes its own steroids in the adrenal gland and these are vital for the body's normal function.

Different types of synthetic steroids have been developed for use in medicine. There is a group called anabolic steroids, which some athletes take (illegally!) to help build up muscle mass and these *should not be confused* with the steroids used in psoriasis.

There is another group called catabolic steroids or glucocorticoids (e.g. prednisolone), which are taken orally (by mouth) because of their anti-inflammatory and immuno-suppressive properties – they damp down the activity of various immune cells in the body that cause inflammation. They are very useful, even life-saving, in some medical conditions such as severe asthma or rheumatoid arthritis. The down side of this group of steroids is that if they are used at a high dose *for a prolonged period* they have many side effects such as weight gain, bone thinning, decreased growth in children, high blood pressure and loss of muscle mass, to name but a few. Because of this down side, doctors try to use these steroids at the lowest possible dose for short periods. This type of oral steroid is used very occasionally in the treatment of a very severe flare-up of psoriasis. However, for the reasons already mentioned, they are normally used for only a few weeks, the starting dose being gradually decreased over this period of time. This method should prevent or minimise any serious side effects.

Fortunately, these anti-inflammatory steroids can also be made into creams or ointments for application directly onto the skin (topical steroids). They act in a similar fashion to their oral counterpart. These creams have been developed to try to produce the same anti-inflammatory properties without all the side effects on the rest of the body, even after long-term use. This approach has been very successful and topical steroids are useful for psoriasis in certain circumstances, in the flexures or if the psoriasis is inflamed.

Why is there so much conflicting information about steroids and their safety?

This is an extremely common question and worry for many people. We are not entirely sure why so much misinformation has been generated about topical steroids but people do seem to have extremely strong views about their safety. The following points may in part explain why some of the myths have developed.

- The very earliest topical steroids developed were poorly regulated and of uncertain strength (potency). Even as late as the early 1980s there was little recognition of the potential danger of excessive use of the potent steroids, and so there were unwanted and undesirable side effects. These included skin thinning if used on skin other than the palms and soles for more than a few weeks. Unfortunately, when this side effect was noticed, topical steroids got a bad name. This bad publicity has regrettably been inappropriately extended, by some people, to all steroids, even the very weak ones. Remember that topical steroids vary enormously in strength. (For examples of steroids, see Appendix 3.)

- Steroids taken by mouth have a number of side effects, and many people assume that topical steroids do as well. This isn't true. Topical steroids were developed specifically to prevent the problems of oral steroids.
- There are different types of steroids. They act differently and have different side effects. It is easy to assume that all steroids are the same and thus misunderstand the side effect risks. For example, *anabolic* steroids can cause an increase in muscle size and liver damage, but this **does not** occur with the topical steroids used in psoriasis.
- Many people have become disillusioned with conventional medicine. There has been a social trend to assume that Western medicines are dangerous and that herbal remedies or natural products are safe and preferable. The word *steroid* has become almost synonymous with all that is bad about conventional medical treatments.
- Steroids do not cure psoriasis, so it often recurs after using them and can 'rebound' (come back) and become worse. You may have expected a cure – partly because the media loves reporting on 'miracle cures' – and might be reluctant to use them again.

We do not claim that any conventional therapy is 100% safe but then neither are less conventional treatments. Risks have to be assessed for any form of therapy. Provided that topical steroids are used appropriately, they are an extremely valuable, safe and effective part of psoriasis therapy. It is interesting that in the USA, where patients are much more likely to sue over adverse effects, dermatologists use more steroid therapy for psoriasis than we do in the UK.

What does 'use sparingly' on my box of steroid ointment mean?

Each box should come with a chart giving details of the correct amount to use, in 'fingertip units'. This indicates the safe and correct amount of steroid to apply by using the last joint of your finger as a way to measure out the steroid. If you are using steroid creams or ointments in a very small area – for example, just under your arms – apply a thin layer and rub it in well.

Vitamin D

My husband's doctor has suggested trying vitamin D treatment. What does this do?

These are topical applications that contain vitamin D derivatives and have been very helpful in the treatment of milder forms of psoriasis. Vitamin D is essential for healthy growth of skin. The topical vitamin D preparations (e.g. Dovonex) are less messy than dithranol and tar, and many people find them very effective. They are available as creams, ointments and scalp applications.

For the treatment to be effective, it is important to apply a 'thick smear' and then gently rub it in. A 'thick smear' means covering the area with cream or ointment so that you can see it on your skin before rubbing it in. Vitamin D does not need to be used 'sparingly', as do steroid creams and ointments, as long as you do not use more than 100g a week.

Should I take a course of vitamin D?

No. Vitamins should be present in a normal healthy diet, and taking supplements will have little or no effect on the skin.

I have noticed that, since I started using this new vitamin D cream, my eyes have become very sore. Is there any link?

This is probably caused by your rubbing your eyes (or even just touching them) after you have applied the vitamin D cream to your body. It is very important that, after applying any of the active treatments, you wash your hands thoroughly to make sure that they are clear of any trace of the treatment. As you have discovered, even the smallest amount can cause irritation when it comes into contact with your face or eyes.

Different treatments for different areas

I have areas of psoriasis on my knees and the doctor has recommended that I use short-contact Dithrocream. I don't really understand what I have to do.

Dithrocream is a type of dithranol that is very helpful in treating well-defined areas of psoriasis, such as those on the elbows and knees. The 'short contact' approach has been designed for use at home. It involves applying gradually increasing strengths of Dithrocream to the plaques of psoriasis and leaving the cream in place for 30 minutes before washing it off (best done in the shower or bath). Apply enough to cover the plaque completely and rub the cream in until it is completely absorbed. Usually the first strength is 0.1%, followed by 0.25%, and goes up to 2%. The Dithrocream must be applied carefully to the plaques, not the good skin, making sure that it doesn't smudge. It should then be washed off after half an hour and moisturisers re-applied. It only needs to be done once a day.

Some people find that the very weak strengths have little or no effect. If this is the case for you, you should move more quickly to the next strength up, spending no more than three or four days at the lower strengths. If you find your skin getting sore, you should either return to a lower strength or discontinue the treatment – it really depends on how sore it is, and this is clearly an individual judgement. To save you money on prescriptions, your GP should prescribe you the five increasing strengths of Dithrocream on one prescription. You would then only have to pay one prescription charge for this.

Micanol is a new formulation of dithranol that can cause less staining if used properly. It comes in strengths of 1% and 3%. If washed off with lukewarm water, Micanol is less likely to stain.

I have psoriasis in the genital area. Can I use the same ointment as I have for my elbows and knees?

In general, your doctor will prescribe different creams for your elbows/knees and for your genital area. The skin in the genital area is thinner and therefore more sensitive than that on your elbows/knees. Using the same treatment there might actually cause damage and soreness. There is also the fact that the genital area tends to be warm and moist, so the treatment is absorbed more readily and therefore does not need to be as strong to be effective. Mild to moderate potency steroids are often used in the genital and other flexural areas (e.g. armpits), and, because infections with yeasts and bacteria are common in these places, are often combined with anti-fungal and anti-bacterial agents.

Which is the best treatment to put on my scalp?

The treatment that you use on your scalp will depend very much on the extent to which it is affected and what you want to achieve.

- **Coconut oil** This is good if your scalp is dry but not necessarily covered with active psoriasis. It is solid at room temperature but melts on contact with the skin and is therefore quite greasy; it has a very light but not unpleasant smell. Use as much as you need to make your scalp feel comfortable.
- **Coal tar solution (Cocois)** If the psoriasis on your scalp is thick and active, this is the best treatment to use, as it moistens the plaques and encourages them to lift off. Because it has tar in it, though, it tends to be a bit messy and has a distinctive smell. The amount you use will depend on how thick your psoriasis is, but apply enough to turn the scale from white to the colour of the ointment.
- **Steroid (e.g. Betnovate) scalp application** This is useful for short-term treatment if your scalp is inflamed but the plaques are not particularly thick. (Beware, though: the scalp application is an alcohol-based solution and can sting when applied.) It is relatively clean and odour free.
- **Vitamin D scalp application** This is useful when the plaques are thin but active. It is clean and odour free. One or two drops are enough to cover an area of your head about the size of a postage stamp.

It is very difficult to apply my scalp treatment. Have you any advice?

With scalp treatment, the method of application is almost as important as which treatment you use. Applying the treatment involves parting the hair in sections and rubbing the treatment along the exposed area. It is best to do this in a sequential fashion, starting at the front of the scalp and working your way round. If the scale/plaques are very thick, once they have been moisturised with the treatment (especially Cocois) they can be gently lifted up using a comb.

It is easier to get someone else to do this for you, as it is difficult to see the top of your head and (a) rub the treatment in where it is needed and (b) lift the scale where appropriate. When doing this some hair may come out, but it will grow back so don't be too perturbed! The best time to do a scalp treatment is before going to bed, because the treatment (especially Cocois and coconut oil) will make your hair look greasy and can smell. Try wearing a cotton 'night cap', a shower cap or something similar and cover your pillows with old pillowcases to protect them. (You can buy pillowcase protectors from bed-linen shops/departments, which give useful extra protection to your pillows.) Wash your hair the next morning with an anti-psoriasis shampoo (i.e. tar-based). An advantage of the coconut-based treatments is that they are wonderful conditioners for your hair!

What can I do treatment-wise to help get rid of psoriasis on my face?

First, apply lots of moisturiser, because this will help keep the scaling under control as well as making your face more comfortable. Often a weak topical steroid will help. Psoriasis on the hairline will respond to a weak coal-tar preparation such as Alphosyl but it is best not to use this type on your face as it can cause discomfort. Tacalcitol (Curatoderm) is also licensed for use on the face. Whichever treatment you use on your face, be very careful not to get any in your eyes.

If the psoriasis on your face does not respond to these treatments, it is worth consulting your doctor again in case there is a fungal or yeast component to the psoriasis (known as seborrhoeic psoriasis). If this is the case, you will need an anti-fungal cream or perhaps an anti-fungal and steroid cream combined.

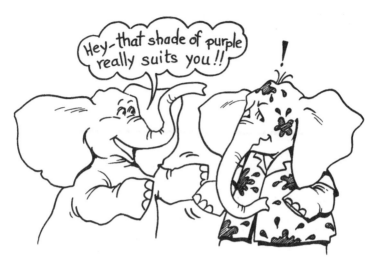

Practical aspects

I have been given Dithrocream, which is making a mess of the bathroom.

It is true that Dithrocream can make a mess of your bathroom, with purple stains. To stop this happening, you need to be very careful not to get the Dithrocream anywhere but on your body. To help to minimise the staining on your bath or shower when you wash it off, you can use cotton wool soaked in baby oil to wipe off the cream before getting into the bath or shower. Just take care not to wipe the Dithrocream onto unaffected skin. If the difficulties you are having with the Dithrocream mean that you are not using the treatment, you need to see your doctor to discuss the possibility of being prescribed another that you do feel able to use.

The scalp lotion I am using is making my forehead so sore. Can I use something else?

You can of course ask your doctor to prescribe something else for your scalp. However, it is worth considering two possible reasons why your forehead is sore. First, are you applying your treatment properly? If you get someone else to do it for you, you may find that they do not get so much on your forehead so it stops being sore. Secondly, try to establish for sure that it is the treatment that is making it sore and not the psoriasis itself. If it is actually the psoriasis that is making your forehead sore, you will need to get a specific treatment for this (a mild steroid or tar application may be appropriate).

Can over-use of a special shampoo (e.g. Polytar) be harmful?

There is no evidence to show that it is. However, it is not sensible to over-use any treatment, so we strongly suggest that you use the shampoo only as often as it recommends on the bottle. Some people report that using the same prescription for a prolonged period makes it less effective. There is no scientific evidence for this except in the case of steroid use.

The skin around the bits where I have psoriasis burns if I get the cream on them. What can I do to stop it?

The first and most obvious thing to say is to be very careful when you apply the cream to ensure that you get it *only* on the plaques. There are two other strategies that might also help.

First, apply a thicker layer of moisturiser around the plaques to protect the skin. This is particularly effective if you are using a thick greasy moisturiser. Apply the moisturiser as you would normally; having allowed the moisturiser to sink in, apply the prescribed topical treatment to the plaques and then carefully apply another thicker layer of moisturiser around each plaque. This is quite time consuming but will be helpful. Secondly, try to minimise the amount of smudging that occurs from the plaque onto the skin that has no psoriasis on it. If you are using a vitamin D cream or a weak tar-based preparation, you can do this by ensuring that you rub the treatment in well and don't put on your clothes until it has been completely absorbed. If you are using short-contact Dithrocream, it is best not to put on any clothes while the Dithrocream is on; if you do put something on, make sure that it is very loose and not going to smudge the cream. The other thing to remember about smudging is that, if you apply a treatment in your groin, under your arms or under your breasts, it may go onto the adjoining unaffected area. The best thing to do in this instance is to make sure that you use a treatment that will not irritate your skin (e.g. a mild topical steroid).

Should I use soap on the areas of psoriasis?

Soap tends to have a drying effect on the skin. The soaps that are advertised as having moisturisers in them are better than others but can still have a drying effect. With this in mind, it is better to find an alternative to soap (i.e. a soap substitute). The one that is often recommended is aqueous cream, which is available from a pharmacist or on prescription, but there are other 'soap substitutes' that you can buy over the counter (e.g. E45 wash). Rather than removing the protective layer of natural oils on your skin as soap does, soap substitutes serve to protect and supplement this. The best way to use them is to have a large pot handy in the bath or shower, to scoop out dollops and rub this over yourself as you might use soap. The cream can then be rinsed off, leaving the skin cleansed and moisturised. If you feel this is not cleansing you adequately in the groin area or under your arms, use small amounts of soap there. It is worth noting that using soap substitutes to wash with should not be seen as a substitute for using a moisturiser once you have had your bath or shower.

Do I have to bandage up the affected skin?

No, you do not have to. Nevertheless, depending on which treatment you are using, covering the skin with tubular bandages (e.g. Tubifast) may be helpful. Particularly if you are using tar-based treatments, these sorts of bandages keep the treatment on your skin, where it should be, and can stop it from getting onto your clothes. Tubular bandages are stretchy cotton bandages that form a sleeve, unlike a normal bandage which needs to be wrapped round. They come in different sizes to fit arms, legs and trunk, and are now available on prescription.

I am breast-feeding my baby daughter and have psoriasis on my breasts. Should I stop using the cream the doctor gave me?

You should make sure, first of all, that you have told your doctor that you are breast-feeding, and he or she will then make sure that anything prescribed is safe for you and your baby. You should also make sure that, whenever you breast-feed, your nipples in particular are clear of any active treatment as this could have a damaging effect on your baby if any gets into her mouth. It is important, however, that you keep the skin on your breasts as supple as possible to prevent cracks forming – especially around the nipples – so you must continue to use your treatment.

Do be aware that, although it is only your nipples that the baby is likely to suck, she will touch the rest of the skin on your breasts. She might therefore come into contact with the topical treatment you have put on – which can be damaging to delicate baby skin. It may be simplest while breast-feeding to stick to moisturisers alone, but do discuss this with your doctor.

Treatments for psoriatic arthropathy

What are the usual treatments for psoriatic arthropathy?

In general, the treatments are the same as for other sorts of arthritis and can be divided into first-line and second-line as with treatment of the skin. The first-line treatments can be started by your GP without the need for specialist advice. In the early stages, it does not matter very much if the diagnosis is not confirmed, because the treatment will be the same for any person with joint pains.

- **Physiotherapy** is often forgotten or used only at later stages of the disease, but can be very useful both to treat pain and stiffness and to educate you about exercises, correct lifting techniques and other simple things that can help prevent further problems.
- **Non-steroidal anti-inflammatory drugs** (NSAIDs) are a class of drugs that were derived from aspirin, and they have a wide range of uses. In arthritis, NSAIDs are used early to relieve pain by working against the inflammation, so they also relieve swelling and stiffness. There are many different brands

and strengths, starting with ibuprofen – which is probably the best known as it was the first one to be made available without prescription, as Nurofen. They have some side effects, of which the most important is irritation of the stomach; this sometimes leads to ulceration, so you should not buy them to use long term without discussing it with your GP. (They are also available as creams and gels to rub directly into the skin over a joint but this is an expensive way of using the drug with little definite evidence that it works.)

- **Steroid injections**. Although steroid tablets should be seen as a second-line treatment, injections directly into a joint can be useful earlier if only one large joint, such as a knee, is affected. Pain relief and getting mobility back can be very rapid, and there is only a risk of the general side effects of steroids if injections are given too often. This should not happen, because other types of treatment would then be indicated. Many GPs are very good at giving steroid injections and will happily do it but others might want to refer you to a specialist if they don't feel confident and have not had much practice in this type of treatment.

5
Second-line treatments

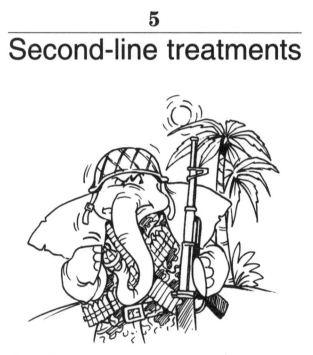

Introduction

The term 'second-line' refers to a treatment that would not be used in the first attempt to treat a patient unless the psoriasis was very severe right from the start. This is usually because the second-line treatment involves attending hospital as either an out-patient or an in-patient, takes up more of the person's time and may have more side effects. There are some very effective treatments that have to be 'held in reserve' in case the disease becomes more widespread or aggressive, as only a limited amount can be used because of their potential side effects. Thus, if one were used for psoriasis that wasn't severe, it might not be an option when it was really needed. Ultra-violet treatment is the best example of this, because the total dose given over a lifetime needs to be limited to minimise the risk of skin cancer.

Although many second-line treatments can produce side effects serious enough to mean that the treatment has to be stopped, all these effects are very well understood. They can be minimised by careful monitoring using blood and other tests, so that treatment is stopped safely before any permanent damage is done. It can therefore be much safer to take a well-researched powerful drug where the dangers are known and understood than some complementary therapies involving herbs where the dangers may be just as great but are not recognised or looked for.

In hospital

I have to go into hospital soon. What sort of treatment may I expect?

To a certain extent, this depends on your consultant and the reasons for your admission to hospital. It is probably reasonable for us to assume that your psoriasis is widespread and causing you a lot of problems, otherwise you wouldn't be admitted. In this case, it is likely that you will be having treatments and investigations. One hospital treatment, called Ingram's method, consists of dithranol paste and ultra-violet (UV) light. Specialist dermatology (skin) nurses will apply the paste to your psoriasis and bandage you up to keep the paste in contact for several hours. When it is removed, you will have UV treatment. This is done once a day and can improve the psoriasis very quickly.

It can be very good for you to have a rest from the daily grind of putting your own treatments on, and some hospitals now have special day therapy units where this can be done for you without the need to be admitted. It is, however, a great problem for some dermatology departments to hang onto their specialist in-patient facilities because hospital managers need to save money and they tend to view skin disease as an out-patient problem. There is nothing more devastating for someone with psoriasis than to be placed in a general medical ward with all sorts of different patients and nurses who lack the special training to deal with your problems. If this applies to your hospital, ask if day care is an alternative, and write to your MP! Self-help groups usually have experience in putting pressure on hospitals and MPs, and should be able to help you phrase a suitable letter.

I recently went into hospital and had the same creams applied to my skin that had failed at home. They worked well – why is this?

If you are admitted to a specialist ward where the staff are properly trained in looking after skin problems, it can be a very restful place. Add to this the chance to relax and avoid any household chores and it is not surprising that treatments work better! You mentioned that creams were applied to your skin – this also makes a difference, as you don't have to worry about finding the time or making sure the creams don't make marks or stains around the house. Many people also enjoy the touching involved, as this can be sadly lacking when you have a skin disease. Some people describe hospital as a place of sanctuary – somewhere safe to escape to – which seems to describe an ideal to be aimed for by all hospitals.

I hate going into hospital to get my psoriasis under control. Is there no alternative?

If you are lucky enough to go to a hospital department with a day-care centre, you can have intensive treatments applied by the nurses and still go to work or back home. It may involve having bandages to cover the creams but is a good alternative if you do not want to stay in hospital or if there are no beds available.

Ultra-violet light treatment

Why is natural sunlight such a good healer?

Natural sunlight is a good healer for many people with psoriasis, but there are some who do not respond and some who are made worse. Sunlight consists of several different types of light across a spectrum ranging from infra-red, through visible light, to ultra-violet (UV). It is the ultra-violet part that can help in treating psoriasis.

The skin cells contain specialised molecules (called chromophores) that are capable of absorbing the energy from UV light and then releasing it to power chemical reactions that affect the function of the cells. In psoriasis, this can result in the cells not multiplying so rapidly and behaving more like normal skin.

Should I buy a sunbed?

'No' is the quick answer to this question! Although ultra-violet (UV) light can help some people with psoriasis and even if you have noticed your skin getting better on holiday, there are dangers in using sunbeds. UV light can lead to the development of skin cancers, and many dermatologists (skin specialists) would advise against anyone using sunbeds. When you have psoriasis, controlled UV treatment can be very effective in clearing your skin, but if you use a sunbed it will be impossible for the hospital to calculate a safe dosage of UV for your skin or for you to be sure that you are getting the right type of UV light.

What is PUVA?

PUVA is a light treatment using a **p**soralen and **UVA**. Natural sunlight contains different types of ultra-violet light labelled 'A' and 'B' (UVA and UVB). UVA on its own is not active in skin disease, but if given with a 'psoralen' (which makes the skin more sensitive to light – photosensitive) it can be very effective. The psoralen, which is derived from plants, is usually taken by mouth but can be applied via a bath containing the chemical, or small areas can be treated using a topical paint. Not all people with psoriasis will benefit from PUVA.

The use of UV light in the UK is governed by guidelines from the British Photodermatology Group, which look at who should be treated and decide on safe total dosages. They have identified three main groups of people who should be considered for PUVA treatment:

- People with severe psoriasis that is not responding to topical treatments.

- People whose psoriasis returns within three to six months of successful treatment as in-patients or in a day centre.
- People who do not want topical treatment and UVB has failed.

How do the doctors know how much UV light to give me?

This is a good question, as we all vary in our reaction to UV light – as you can see on any beach in the summer! The dose of UV light used in PUVA is worked out from the lowest amount that will turn your type of skin red. This is known as the 'minimum erythema dose' (erythema meaning 'redness of the skin'). The redness lasts for 48–72 hours, so treatment is usually given twice a week to allow the skin to recover between doses. As you progress through a course of PUVA the dose is slowly increased to compensate for the tanning effect, which starts to block some of the UV light.

Why can't I continue having PUVA to keep my skin clear?

UV radiation causes skin damage and, eventually, skin cancer, and doctors have to be very careful not to put you at unnecessary risk. After a total of 200 sessions of PUVA your risk of developing skin cancer (other than the serious melanoma-type cancer) would have increased tenfold. Sessions are usually limited to between 150 and 200 but even then you would need careful follow-up once a year to check your skin for early signs of cancer.

As well as the overall maximum, it is recommended that you have no more than 30 sessions in any one year. So it would be a shame to use up your 'allowance' to keep your skin clear and not be able to use it if the psoriasis came back. Using the total number of sessions as a guide is better than looking at the total dose (measured in joules per square centimetre of skin) because the dose varies according to your type of skin. An average 'white' British skin type might mean a total dose of 1000–1500 joules per square centimetre as the equivalent of 150–200 sessions.

Why do I need to wear sunglasses on the days I have PUVA?

Because most people take the psoralen by mouth, it affects more than just the skin. The eyes are also made more sensitive to light, which can cause cataracts to develop. To protect your eyes, you must wear glasses that filter out the UV rays. These need to be worn for the rest of the day. If you feel uncomfortable wearing sunglasses all day, you can get spectacles with clear glass that filters out UV light, but make absolutely certain they are the right type.

Some people are very nauseated by the drug and are, therefore, sometimes treated with psoralen by lying in a solution of it in a bath before the UVA treatment. Even then, enough of the drug may be absorbed into the body to make the eyes sensitive and at risk, so sunglasses are still needed.

I have had PUVA treatment but it seems that my psoriasis has got worse. Why is this?

There might be a couple of ways to explain this. Most patients with psoriasis can be helped by UV treatment but some are not and some get worse. Usually this is obvious from the pattern of your psoriasis: if you get worse in summer and better in winter, extra UV light is not for you. The other explanation would depend on the severity of your psoriasis. If it is bad and going through a natural cycle of getting worse, any treatment might seem to fail.

If you mean that your psoriasis improved or cleared with PUVA and then recurred in a more severe form later on, there is unlikely to be a link with the treatment.

Why do doctors offer treatments like PUVA with a slight risk involved when the end result isn't very good?

PUVA and its risks are very well understood and for most people it can work well, clearing the skin and delaying the return of psoriasis. All patients having PUVA are carefully counselled about the risks and most of them agree that they are acceptable. Most of the risk is from the UV light but in some circumstances the psoralen can cause problems. If there is a chance of damage to the liver from causes such as heavy drinking or because of a history of jaundice, the psoralen can cause extra damage. In such instances, blood tests are needed to make sure that the liver is working normally before using the treatment. Psoriasis is a tricky condition to treat because it can vary in its response to treatment – not just between people but also between different attacks in the same person. You might not respond well to PUVA on one occasion but it could work better in the future. Because of this variation, we need as many different ways of treating people as possible.

It is also very useful to be able to use treatments such as PUVA to give people a break from the daily grind of applying creams. We once heard a consultant describe his patients as being 'war weary' from the constant battle with their psoriasis.

In studies of people's attitudes to psoriasis and the risk of treatments, many patients preferred to take a tablet with some side effects if it worked and cleared their psoriasis. The general comment was that to live to 65 with no psoriasis would be a lot better than to live to 75 with psoriasis!

I have been offered narrow band UVB treatment. What does this mean?

UVB contains quite a wide range of wavelengths, and although it can be useful in guttate psoriasis, it has never been as useful as PUVA for other types. In the last few years, a more defined form of UVB has been developed – hence the name 'narrow band'. This seems to be almost as effective as PUVA without all the drawbacks of taking the psoralen. It may also carry less risk of causing skin cancer in the long term, although this will necessarily take a long time to evaluate properly. Like PUVA, the aim of treatment is to clear the skin and this can be achieved by having three treatments a week for between five and eight weeks.

Methotrexate

My wife's doctor has prescribed methotrexate. Is it a steroid?

No, methotrexate (MTX) is a drug that acts to stop rapid or excessive cell growth – a 'cytotoxic' agent. It stops the rapid turnover of skin cells that cause the typical plaques of psoriasis. Unfortunately, it doesn't just act on the skin, so care has to be taken to prevent damage to other organs, especially the liver.

I have heard that methotrexate is a drug originally developed for the treatment of cancer. If so, is there any connection between the two conditions, and is the effect of methotrexate the same in both conditions?

There is no connection between the two conditions in that neither is more common if you suffer from the other. Both psoriasis and cancer, however, involve cells growing and multiplying more rapidly than they should, so the 'cytotoxic' action of methotrexate has the same effect on those cells. It can be used because cells that are growing normally are not as sensitive to the drug as the abnormal ones.

I take methotrexate and understand it can affect the liver. Are there any long-term problems from taking this drug?

Damage to the liver can occur with long-term use of methotrexate but it can also affect the bone marrow and interfere with the production of blood cells. The drug tends to be used in low doses in psoriasis, so it doesn't cause many other problems. In the higher doses used in some cancer treatments (chemotherapy) it can have toxic effects on the lungs and gut.

Why do I have to have a liver biopsy – wouldn't a blood test be enough?

Methotrexate can damage the liver and, because the side effects are well known, doctors like to be able to minimise or prevent them. If you waited for signs of liver damage to show up in the blood you might have developed long-term problems. The liver biopsy, which involves using a wide needle to take a small sample of the liver tissue, can show some very early and subtle changes before they do you any harm. There are, of course, some risks in having a liver biopsy, and you usually need to spend a day in hospital in case of internal bleeding; this added risk is taken into consideration when weighing up the pros and cons of using the treatment. Liver biopsies are not done very often, maybe only every couple of years depending on the dose you need.

Recent research has suggested that a blood test for a substance called 'pro-collagen 3' may be able to indicate the presence of any liver damage accurately enough to prevent the need for a liver biopsy. The test should soon be generally available.

Does methotrexate interfere with other drugs?

There are some problems with methotrexate and other drugs you may be prescribed or buy over the counter which tend to make the methotrexate more toxic. The common drugs are trimethoprim (an antibiotic), phenytoin (a drug for epilepsy), aspirin and other anti-inflammatory drugs such as ibuprofen, some 'water' tablets (diuretics) used to treat blood pressure and heart failure, and the retinoid drugs such as Neotigason (mentioned below).

I am doing very well on methotrexate, as it keeps my skin almost clear. Why do I have to keep going to the hospital for a prescription?

Although methotrexate can be prescribed by GPs, it is a drug that they do not have to use very often. This means that they may not be happy to take the responsibility of prescribing it, in case errors are made or they do not spot any potential problems. We know of at least one case where a GP's repeat prescription gave a daily dose rather than a weekly one, which could have caused severe problems for the patient. Many GPs do prescribe methotrexate but it is still a good idea to have a regular review in the hospital as well. It might be worth asking your GP to prescribe it so that you do not have to attend the hospital so often.

Does having taken methotrexate in the past affect my chances of getting pregnant?

This depends on how long ago you took the drug. It does affect the rate of production of eggs in women and of sperm in men, so it should be stopped for three months before you start trying for a baby, to allow this effect to wear off.

Vitamin A

I've read that vitamin A treatment is good. What is it all about?

Otherwise known as retinoids, vitamin-A-derived treatments can be very helpful with moderate to severe psoriasis. Neotigason (acitretin) is the drug name that you are most likely to encounter. There are a number of side (unwanted) effects with this class of drug, as well as some circumstances when it should not be used. Because it is teratogenic (it damages the unborn child), it should be given only in exceptional circumstances to women of child-bearing age. It can also cause nausea, dryness of the mucous membranes (mainly the eyes and lips) and temporary hair loss. A cream derived from vitamin A has recently become available (Zorac; tazarotene) and is a useful addition to the treatments on offer although it can also cause dryness and irritation of the skin.

Should I take a course of vitamin A?

No. Vitamins should be present in a normal healthy diet, and taking supplements will have little or no effect on the skin. Vitamin A in particular is harmful if taken to excess, especially if you are pregnant.

I have been taking Neotigason tablets for two years and now I am thinking of trying for a baby. How long will I have to wait before the effects have worn off?

Neotigason is a retinoid drug derived from vitamin A and is very useful in some forms of psoriasis. Unfortunately, it can lead to severe deformities in a developing baby, so you must not take it when pregnant. The drug persists in the body in very small amounts for a long time and, as this would be enough to cause the damage, you should wait for two years after stopping treatment before trying for a baby.

We hope that this was explained to you before you started the treatment. It is good practice for doctors to ask women to sign a consent form before starting the drug, to show that they have been given, and have understood, a full explanation of the effects and the absolute need for contraceptive precautions.

My husband is taking Neotigason. Is it safe for us to try for a baby?

Although Neotigason can harm developing babies, it does not affect the production of sperm and does not cause changes to the genetic material. So it is safe for you to try for a baby.

My consultant has offered me PUVA as well as Neotigason, as the latter hasn't worked on its own. Isn't this risky?

Treatment using a retinoid (Neotigason) and **PUVA** is called RePUVA. The combination works quite well but is usually reserved for difficult cases – such as when there is little improvement after 50 PUVA treatments, or the psoriasis returns within six months of successful PUVA treatment or there is severe psoriasis on the palms and soles. The advantages of using this combination are that the retinoid can decrease the total amount of UV exposure needed and also acts to prevent some of the skin changes that might lead to cancer.

Cyclosporin

Why have I been offered treatment with cyclosporin? I have a friend who takes this because he has had a kidney transplant.

The use of cyclosporin reflects the importance of your immune system in the psoriatic process. It is a drug that is used to alter the body's immune response and hence helps prevent rejection of transplants. A transplant patient with psoriasis noticed that the psoriasis improved dramatically with the cyclosporin, and it was tried with success in non-transplant patients. It has an effect on only part of the immune system, specifically suppressing a chemical called interleukin-2, so does not increase the risks of infection in the way that other immune-suppressing drugs (e.g. steroids) do. There are some concerns about a possible increased risk of developing cancer after long-term treatment, so careful follow-up is usually advised even after treatment has ended.

I have to have my blood pressure checked regularly because I take cyclosporin. Why is this?

Like all drugs, cyclosporin has side effects and the main problems are possible kidney damage and high blood pressure. Both of these unwanted effects are reversible (i.e. kidney function and blood pressure will return to normal) if they are detected early, so regular monitoring is essential. We hope that you are also having regular blood tests to look at your kidney function. Often the blood pressure rises a little with this drug, but as long as your kidneys are OK you can continue with the treatment. It can be so successful that patients are reluctant to stop it, so occasionally an additional drug can be given to control the blood pressure without long-term risks.

There are a number of lesser side effects that can be a great nuisance. These include pins and needles in the fingers, a mild tremor (shaking or trembling) and nausea, but these usually occur early in treatment and improve if it is continued. More troublesome can be extra hair growth and enlargement of the gums. The former can be very upsetting for women, who may stop treatment because of it. The latter is more common if dental hygiene is poor, so it can be minimised with regular visits to the dentist.

My doctor says that taking cyclosporin can make it difficult to treat other conditions. Why is this?

Cyclosporin interacts with a number of oral treatments but not with topical ones. This interaction means that the side effects of cyclosporin are more likely to occur or that it may not work at all. You must tell any doctor who is treating you that you are taking cyclosporin, as there is a long list of problem drugs. Avoid buying over-the-counter drugs in shops where there is no pharmacist to advise you, and don't take herbal or other remedies for which the effects are unknown. The common problem drugs are:

- **antibiotics** erythromycin (a common antibiotic) should be avoided, but penicillin is safe;
- **pain killers** aspirin and related drugs, including ibuprofen (Advil, Brufen and Nurofen) and mefenamic acid (Ponstan), should be avoided, but paracetamol is safe;

- **anti-malarials** chloroquine can interact with other drugs, so avoid it if you are travelling abroad.

Treatments for psoriatic arthropathy

The usual treatments don't seem to be helping my psoriatic arthropathy. What other treatments are there?

As with skin psoriasis, this is where second-line treatments or disease-modifying drugs are used. This indicates that the drugs alter the disease itself rather than dealing with the effects of the disease – in this case the inflammation.

- **Methotrexate** is also used for other types of arthritis, so it fits in well if you have skin and joint psoriasis. It has been dealt with earlier in this chapter, where the dosages and precautions are discussed. It is taken as a small weekly dose and needs careful monitoring.
- **Steroids** are powerful anti-inflammatory drugs, so can have a dramatic effect in treating an acute flare-up of arthritis. In some cases they are also used long term in low doses to try to keep a balance between benefit and the potential side effects listed in the section *Steroids* in Chapter 4. If steroids are used in high doses, careful monitoring of the skin psoriasis is essential because rapid changes in steroid dose can cause problems, with dramatic worsening of the skin sometimes to the point of pustular psoriasis or erythroderma (discussed in Chapter 2).
- **Other agents**. Immuno-suppressive drugs such as azathioprine and cyclosporin are sometimes used but seem to be less effective for the arthritis. Occasionally, sulfasalazine (Salazopyrin) is used. This is another type of anti-inflammatory drug that is often taken for inflammatory gut disease such as ulcerative colitis. Some people with ulcerative colitis can get a type of arthritis in the lower back; they noted that the arthritis improved with treatment of their gut problems. It was then used for other forms of arthritis and has become a useful back-up drug if people cannot tolerate the more usual treatments.

- **Gold injections** are used less often than they were in the past for all forms of arthritis. They were used only rarely for psoriatic arthropathy, because one of the common side effects is a skin rash! In a few patients they have worked well and so might be considered if all else fails.

I have just started on methotrexate for my joints but it hasn't helped yet. Can I still take some ibuprofen?

The answer is 'Yes' – but carefully and after discussion with your specialist. Ibuprofen and similar non-steroidal anti-inflammatory drugs do act (interact) with methotrexate, because they alter the way the body gets rid of it. This tends to raise the level of methotrexate in your body and thus increases the chance of side effects, but in the early stages of treatment you are likely to be on a low dose so this will not be so important. Rheumatologists tend to be more relaxed than dermatologists are about the two drugs being used together, as they see the benefits of improved mobility and less pain for their patients. Once again, it is a question of discussing your own situation with your doctor and weighing up the benefits against the possible risks.

I have joint and skin problems with my psoriasis and wonder if I should see a different specialist as well as my dermatologist.

This depends on several things. The most important is how bad your joint problems are, because the worse they are, the more helpful it would be for you to see a rheumatologist – the name for a specialist in joint problems. Some dermatologists become expert in treating psoriatic arthropathy and can certainly start some of the second-line treatment mentioned above. Some hospitals have combined clinics where dermatologists and rheumatologists work together; we think this is an ideal setting to help you if you have both severe psoriasis and severe arthritis.

Other treatments

I have heard that lasers can be used to treat psoriasis. Is this available on the NHS?

Laser treatment of psoriasis is still being researched and evaluated, so is not freely available on the NHS at present. If it proves successful, it should be available within a few years, especially as the cost of laser equipment is coming down. One early approach was to remove the plaques with a laser but this was unsuccessful. Better results seem to come from tuning a laser to destroy the blood vessels feeding the plaques but the more likely use of lasers lies in treatments similar in nature to PUVA. Lasers are capable of activating chemicals applied to plaques so that they directly affect the disease process itself. As you can guess, this still will not provide a cure but could be a useful and safe alternative to UV light.

Antibiotics help with infections. Would they help my psoriasis?

In general, no. The only type of psoriasis that can be helped by antibiotics is the guttate form where the trigger has been a throat infection caused by the bacterium *Streptococcus*. A toxin produced by the bacterium is the cause in these cases and, even if the throat seems better, it is worth taking a course of an antibiotic to ensure that the bacterium is eradicated so that no further toxin is produced to cause the psoriatic reaction.

Using creams is so messy and time consuming. Why can't I take pills instead?

This is a good question but one that is very difficult to answer as we don't know any details of your psoriasis. In general, creams and ointments are safer than pills because the actions can be limited to the skin. The side effects of pills are well known to doctors and, when deciding on the best treatment for you, they have to balance the side effects with any possible benefit. If your psoriasis is very bad or widespread, this balance is in favour of tablets, but if the psoriasis is less widespread, it can be a difficult decision. We feel that patients should be very much involved in

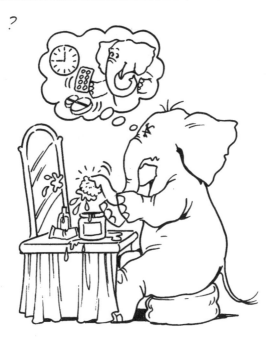

making this type of decision, as they are the ones 'doing' the treating.

Creams can be messy and time consuming and have 'side effects' on quality of life, so it is very tempting to look at different types of treatment. The daily routine of applying creams can be tedious, even with psoriasis that affects only a little of the total skin area, and sometimes people need a break. This can be achieved by using tablets or other non-cream treatments for a short while.

None of the simple treatments has helped my nails. What can I do to improve them?

The treatment of nails is very difficult. You should keep them short to prevent further damage from catching them, and ask your doctor about having the clippings analysed to make sure you do not have a fungal infection. A fungal infection can be an additional problem in damaged nails but can also mimic the typical changes of psoriasis. Topical vitamin D agents on the affected part can sometimes work if applied and covered with polythene, but this may only be practical at night. Other treatments include injecting the growing part of your nail with a steroid, or using some of the tablet treatments. Nails do sometimes improve if the rest of your psoriasis clears up.

6
Complementary therapy

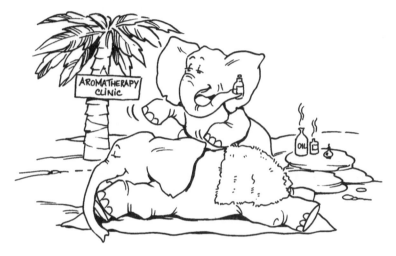

Introduction

These days almost all health books for patients or their families or carers need to contain a section on complementary or 'non-conventional' treatments. These used to be referred to as 'alternative' but, as many of them are becoming more accepted and regulated, they are best thought of as 'complementary' to reflect the fact that they can sit alongside conventional treatments rather than replacing them. Although there is no scientific evidence that, for example, aromatherapy or reflexology is effective in treating psoriasis itself, they are often very helpful in making you feel better and more relaxed.

A whole range of different approaches to helping you with your psoriasis are available outside the NHS, and many practitioners are genuinely trying to improve the quality of life of their clients. It is true to say, however, that there are also some people and clinics who make exaggerated claims for their particular approach or product. There is little regulation of this activity, although a recent report from the All Party Parliamentary Group on Skin has looked at what can or should be done to help protect consumers by using existing Trading Standards legislation or by introducing new powers for the Medicines Control Agency.

A wealth of information is available on all sorts of different ways to treat psoriasis and we are sure that there are many new treatments awaiting discovery or proper evaluation. It is the evaluation that makes this chapter very difficult to write. People who get better from complementary treatment are always very positive about it, as are the practitioners, and you will very rarely find anyone advertising the fact that a treatment has failed to work or made them worse. Most of the success stories are what we would call 'anecdotal evidence' – based on what people have reported on how they have found relief – and a lot of anecdotes are needed to make a proven case. Proper scientific studies are needed to fully evaluate different therapies and to prove their safety. It may not matter if a person chooses to spend money on a treatment that doesn't work, but it does matter if it makes them worse or ill in some other way. Every year we hear reports of people dying from toxic effects of herbal remedies, both Chinese and Western, so great care is needed in choosing a complementary practitioner.

Many 'miracle cures' seem to be advertised direct to the public now. Some of these have been found to contain undeclared potent steroids, and we recommend extreme caution before you buy or use anything without first taking advice from a doctor or recognised complementary practitioner.

Choosing a safe practitioner

Most complementary practitioners work privately and are better than NHS doctors at 'selling' their treatment. They also tend to spend more time with patients and there is undoubted benefit in being able to talk about your psoriasis and its impact on you. It can be very relaxing to talk, and we wish the NHS system could allow more time than it does for consultations. This is not to say that the only benefit from complementary medicine comes from spending money to buy 'protected time'. It is worth remembering that the term 'complementary' is used deliberately instead of 'alternative', as these treatments should sit alongside the standard first-line treatments (discussed in Chapter 4) and not replace them.

There are now professional bodies that regulate most forms of complementary treatment and you should contact them before choosing a practitioner. Remember that people do not need any medical qualifications to work in complementary medicine, so discuss your plans with your GP so that you can at least check if the practitioner gets the diagnosis right.

The Royal College of Nursing has put together some very sensible guidelines for you to use when choosing a safe practitioner:

• What are the practitioner's qualifications and how long was the training?
• Is he/she a member of a recognised, registered body with a code of practice?
• Can he/she give you the name, address and telephone number of this body so you can check?
• Is the therapy available on the NHS?
• Can your GP delegate care to the practitioner? *[This usually happens only with a referral to a homoeopathic hospital.]*
• Does he/she keep your GP informed?
• Is this the most suitable complementary therapy for your psoriasis?
• Are the records confidential?
• What is the likely total cost of treatment?
• How many treatments will be needed?
• What insurance cover does the practitioner have if things go wrong?

Then ask yourself the following questions:

- Did the practitioner answer your questions clearly and to your satisfaction?
- Did he/she give you written information to look through at your leisure?
- Did the practitioner conduct him/herself in a professional manner?
- Were excessive claims made about the treatment?

You should avoid anyone who:

- Claims to be able to completely cure psoriasis.
- Advises you to stop your conventional treatment without consulting your GP.
- Makes you feel uncomfortable – you need a good relationship if you are going to get full benefit from the treatment.

In short, you should demand the same standards from the practitioner as you would from an NHS doctor and give the claims the same critical scrutiny that is increasingly applied to NHS treatment.

Aromatherapy

Is it safe to have an aromatherapy massage with psoriasis?

Yes it is, if the massage is confined to normal skin. Massage can be very relaxing and this can help you cope with having psoriasis. You should avoid having any large plaques massaged, because the friction and oils may irritate the skin. Areas where the skin is simply dry will benefit from the moisturising effect of the oils. As with other techniques that involve touch, this in itself can be very enjoyable if you find that other people tend to be reluctant to touch you when they see your psoriasis.

Reflexology

What is reflexology, and can it help?

Reflexology is a massage therapy that uses acupuncture points on the feet that represent different parts of the body. The feet are massaged with talcum powder and you don't need to take off any other clothes if you are self-conscious about your skin. Again, the physical contact can be beneficial and it is another good way to relax and feel more able to cope with having psoriasis. This, in itself, seems able to influence the disease, as a positive attitude can help your body fight it.

Chinese herbs

Chinese medicine is said to have made great advances towards helping the disease by looking at it as a whole body problem and using herbs to adjust the balance. How successful is this? Will it become available on the NHS?

Chinese herbal treatments come in two main forms – creams and preparations taken by mouth. (Some other forms are used occasionally, such as bath additives.) It is most common to take preparations by mouth, and this has undergone some trial work by traditional doctors. There seems to be some evidence that certain formulas can be beneficial in psoriasis but research studies have been quite small scale and need further evaluation. It is unlikely that it will become available on the NHS in the foreseeable future, as the testing of drugs and similar items before they are allowed to be prescribed takes many years and is very expensive. This is necessary to try to exclude any products that might have dangerous short- or long-term side effects.

Bear in mind that:

- There is no evidence that Chinese herbs cure psoriasis but there may be some benefits for some people.
- Chinese herbs are not always safe, as they can cause inflammation of and damage to internal organs such as the

liver and kidneys in the short term. The long-term side effects are not known.

- The raw ingredients or herbs are not under any form of quality control, so the chemical composition can vary enormously. The country of origin, the time of year picked and the storage of the herbs can all have an effect on quality.
- There is a similar lack of control over the 'doctors' who sell the herbs. They are not medically qualified Western doctors under the control of the General Medical Council. Many are responsible people but you must remember that anyone can sell these herbs. A lot of money can be made when you consider that costs can be £20–£30 per patient per week.

Recent reports ranging from undeclared potent steroids in Chinese herbal creams to deaths from kidney failure from treatments taken by mouth have highlighted the potential dangers of these preparations. There are calls for better regulation and more research, which are echoed by the reputable practitioners themselves. In the next few years we may be able to recommend a range of herbal treatments, but at present we would caution against them.

Other herbal remedies

Are there any non-Chinese herbal remedies?

Yes, there is a strong tradition of Western herbal medicine, with its origins going back into folklore. Unfortunately, there seems to be even less published work in this area, so very little evidence exists on which someone with a conventional approach can base advice. Herbalists do spend time taking a good medical history and tend to use creams that can be soothing and act as a good emollient, if nothing else.

Many of our modern remedies have been produced after the study of traditional plant-based remedies, but an active ingredient needs to be identified and thoroughly tested before it can be licensed as a drug. This method may well ignore the beneficial effects of groups of extracts that, on their own, may be ineffective but which work well together.

What is *Mahonia aquifolium*?

This is a plant otherwise known as the Oregon grape. Extracts have traditionally been used to treat a variety of conditions, of which psoriasis is one. It is applied in an ointment, and some studies have suggested that it can help some patients. Although the way it works is not known, it might merit further investigation.

Homoeopathy

I have a friend who sees a homoeopathic doctor instead of an ordinary GP. I don't know anything about homoeopathy – would it help my psoriasis?

Homoeopaths believe that the symptoms of a disease are actually the body's way of fighting the disease. They try to help this reaction by using minute doses of a substance that would normally produce the same symptoms if it were used in a higher dose in a healthy person. This 'remedy' is produced by multiple dilutions so that no more than a trace of the substance is present, and the resulting treatment is usually safe and free from side effects. It is very difficult to know whether you could benefit, because psoriasis is not one of the diseases that homoeopathy has been shown to help consistently – unlike, for example, eczema.

Is it expensive to see a homoeopath?

It might be free, as homeopathy is one of the complementary treatments you can have on the NHS. There are five homoeopathic hospitals in Britain – Bristol, Glasgow, Liverpool, London and Tunbridge Wells – staffed by medically qualified doctors who are often local GPs with special qualifications. It is between you and your GP as to whether you can be referred, so if it is not possible, or you feel it is too far to travel, you could see someone privately at a cost of around £20–£30 per consultation. You do not need a prescription for homoeopathic remedies. Some pharmacists have qualifications in homoeopathy and could advise you if you wanted to buy one to try. Contact the Society of Homoeopathy or the British Homoeopathic Association (addresses in Appendix 1) for more information and a list of recognised practitioners in your area.

Other approaches

Does hypnotherapy work at all?

It may help by relaxing you and giving you a more positive approach to the disease, making it easier for you to cope with. It seems to work well if your skin is very itchy, as it can help you to scratch less. Scratching an itch is often pleasurable and you can get locked into a cycle of itching and scratching and itching and so on. Hypnotherapy can help to break this cycle and give your skin a chance to rest. We don't know of any worthwhile studies that show that it directly helps the psoriasis itself, though.

A lot has been said about the Dead Sea and its benefits, and I understand that some countries such as Germany will help towards the cost of treatment there. Would it not make more sense for the NHS to pay for patients to go there rather than pay for expensive drug treatment here?

This is an attractive but rather over-simplified view. The combination of the concentrated salt solution that is the Dead Sea and strong sunshine does seem to be of benefit but the precise mechanism has not been fully evaluated. The sea water also contains some tars that may also be of benefit. Holidays in sunny places can be relaxing and if other people with psoriasis are at the same resort you would be much less afraid to take your clothes off and expose your skin, thus getting more benefit from the sun. As the Dead Sea is below sea level, the atmosphere is relatively thicker and absorbs some of the UVB

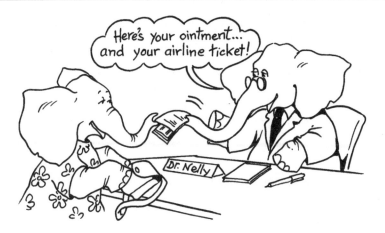

light that causes burning. This means that you can get a higher concentration of the helpful UVA light without burning, but this could lead to higher risks from skin cancer. Most of the reviews of Dead Sea treatment mention treatment times of under three hours. It is thought that the complex salt solution adds to the efficacy of natural sunlight and may in itself have some effect on skin cell turnover. Even the dermatologists from the Ben Gurion University in Israel stress that treatment guidelines and standards have to be set in order to assess the cost effectiveness of Dead Sea therapy compared with other treatments.

The NHS has to be very careful about spending money in this way, and many other patients might demand holidays because they feel better afterwards. One of us has asthma and it always improves on holiday, away from pollution etc. Does this mean that the NHS should pay for a holiday?!

I saw an advert for Dead Sea mud. Could this save me the cost of a trip to Israel?

You will probably be wasting your money. Dark mud seems to help with absorption of UV light and can be useful as a mud pack on painful joints to help increase circulation. However, this is probably not specific to the type of mud found around the Dead Sea and sold in the UK.

Dead Sea bath salts should probably be looked at in the same way. As mentioned in the previous answer, they may have a beneficial effect when combined with the UV light around the Dead Sea but on their own there is little evidence to make the product worth buying.

Is it true that special bathing pools in Turkey can cure psoriasis?

No. I think you are referring to the 'fish that treat psoriasis' as featured in the national press some years ago. There are fish in Turkish bathing pools that nibble away the plaques of psoriasis but they certainly don't cure it! Removing the plaques does allow treatment to reach the underlying skin more easily and this includes sunlight, so the psoriasis may well clear for a while but is just as likely to recur.

How can I find out more about the products advertised in newspapers?

A useful source of information is an American website called the 'Psoriasis Hall of Pshame' (www.pinch.com/skin/pshame. html). It welcomes comments about unusual claims for treatments and reviews the latest advertisements for you to make up your own mind about them.

7
Children and psoriasis

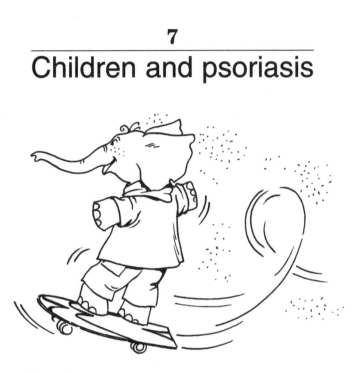

Introduction

Although psoriasis is much less common in childhood than other skin problems such as eczema, about 10% of adults with psoriasis seem to have developed it before the age of 10. If children do have it, the average age when it started (age of onset) is 8 years and, unlike adults where there is no difference between men and women, girls are more likely to have psoriasis than are boys. Some studies have put this difference as high as two to one. There are other differences in that the rash may not appear in the same patterns as with adults, although 65% of children still have the typical distribution of large psoriatic plaques over the knees, elbows and lower back. Guttate and scalp psoriasis are more common in childhood, as is psoriasis in the napkin area and flexures (e.g. groin, armpit, behind the knee). This latter type of psoriasis is the commonest form when infants are affected and is often mistaken for a more straightforward nappy rash.

Because children are not just small adults, management of their psoriasis must take into account certain factors:

- Both the child and his or her parents need educating about the disease.
- The wishes of the parents and the child may be different in respect of the aims of treatment.
- The psychological effects on the child must not be overlooked.
- There are higher risks to children from the absorption of certain creams.
- Because there is a lack of medical research on their effects on children, many treatments are actually not licensed for use in childhood. This needs to be properly discussed before parents consent to treatment for their child.

Babies and psoriasis

My baby has a bright red rash under his nappy. I have psoriasis and worry that he has it as well.

Rashes in the napkin area can be very confusing but psoriasis is quite likely if the rash is bright red. Under a nappy and in the skin creases around the bottom, psoriasis does not show scales, so it does look red and glistening. It will be very clearly demarcated – i.e. it will be very obvious where the rash stops and normal skin takes over.

My baby has psoriasis. I thought only old people got it.

Psoriasis can occur for the first time in people of any age but your baby is unlucky, as it is relatively rare in young children. It most commonly 'presents' (appears first) between the ages of 10 and 40, with some peaks at times of bodily changes such as puberty and the menopause.

Childhood infections

My 7-year-old daughter had guttate psoriasis after a throat infection. Should she have her tonsils removed?

If she has had only one attack, the answer is 'No'. There is some evidence that having their tonsils removed (tonsillectomy) does reduce the number of severe attacks of guttate psoriasis in children who get it frequently or reduces flare-ups in plaque psoriasis. On its own, however, having psoriasis is not a reason to have her tonsils taken out.

My daughter has been told that she has tinea amiantacea in her scalp. I thought 'tinea' was a medical word for ringworm – has she got this as well as psoriasis?

Your daughter does have psoriasis in the scalp, and in children the build-up of scale can be dramatic, coating the hair and causing hair loss. However, any hair loss will not be permanent, as the underlying psoriasis does not scar the skin or damage hair follicles. The name is confusing and reflects the fact that the first doctors to label it felt that it was caused by ringworm; it is one of several inappropriate names for skin diseases that have persisted despite better understanding of their cause.

Children and steroids

My daughter has a lot of psoriasis and it responds very well to steroid creams but our GP is reluctant to prescribe them. Can I insist that he does?

Your GP is obviously well aware of the risks of using steroids in young children. All but the mildest should be avoided if at all possible, especially if a large area of skin needs treating. Children's skin allows for much easier absorption of drugs than does adults' skin, and this is made more of a problem by the size of children. They have more skin surface area for absorption in relation to their total body size compared with adults, so greater care is needed when using creams that can act throughout the body. Steroids applied to the skin can be absorbed in high enough concentrations to have the same side effects as though they were taken by mouth. You need to listen to your GP, and he needs to be able to offer you an alternative treatment or an opportunity to visit a hospital specialist.

Children and psoriatic arthropathy

My 4-year-old daughter has a swollen knee and one painful finger, and the consultant looking after her thinks it is because I have psoriasis. Does this mean I have caused her psoriasis?

You have absolutely nothing to feel guilty about, and we are sorry to hear that you have been worried. There are some forms of arthritis that affect young children, and one of these is called *juvenile psoriatic arthritis*. The skin form of the psoriasis is uncommon in children, so the rash may not be seen for many years. The arthritis tends not to affect very many joints, is not symmetrical and can affect both small and large joints, so your daughter's seemingly odd 'presentation' with a knee and a finger affected would have suggested psoriasis as a possible cause. Because you have psoriasis, this diagnosis is more likely, as your daughter has probably inherited the tendency in the same way that you did. You had no control over this!

We are glad to learn that your daughter has a consultant looking after her, as this type of childhood arthritis can be quite troublesome and last longer than similar types where there is no suspicion of psoriasis.

I have talked to other parents at the out-patient arthritis clinic my daughter goes to, and some of them have to take their children to an eye specialist as well. Should I arrange this for my daughter?

It can be confusing talking to other parents, as you probably take your daughter to a clinic for children with lots of different types of arthritis. Although the psoriatic type can be more troublesome, some of the other types may have more serious complications. One of these, called uveitis, has inflammation in the eye that can cause blindness – hence the need for regular eye checks. Although it occurs only rarely in psoriatic arthritis, it is worth asking your daughter's consultant about it.

School problems

The teacher says my son can't go to school. What should I do?

If your son's teacher is excluding him from school because of his psoriasis, this is a serious problem. You must talk to the teacher and head to establish exactly what the difficulty is. Your GP, the school nursing service, the local community paediatrician and your consultant will be able to help you. There are no grounds for excluding children who have psoriasis, and your school needs help to understand the disease and not to be afraid of it.

8
Feelings, family and friends

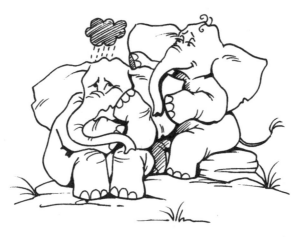

Introduction

The psychological impact of almost any disease is very important. This is especially true for psoriasis where not only the appearance of the plaques but also the consequence of the showers of scales that can come off need to be taken into account. Staying at other people's homes or even trying on clothes in a shop can be very difficult because of the fear of leaving scales behind. The effect on each individual will vary, but not in a simple way; it is not just linked to the severity of the disease. People will respond in different ways and the disease will have a whole range of impacts on individuals' lives. There is no right and wrong way to respond, and no one should feel guilty for experiencing very negative feelings in relation to their psoriasis.

People with psoriasis do not live in isolation, so the disease affects not only them but also their family, loved ones and friends. The aim of the advice offered in this chapter is to encourage you to live as normal a life as possible (bearing in mind that 'normal' is different for each individual), using the help and support of those around you. Because each person and their family and friends are different, it is not always easy to give straightforward answers to questions about coping and about the feelings associated with having psoriasis. In this chapter we offer advice that has been helpful for many of the people we have come into contact with.

Relationships

I have just met a girl I really like, but I don't want her to find out I've got psoriasis. What do other people say?

People handle these situations in different ways. However, we would say that if you think this relationship is likely to last you should tell your girlfriend that you have psoriasis. There are two reasons for this. First, she is likely to notice the plaques – especially if you become intimate. Second and more important, you will probably feel better/more relaxed once you have told her. Although it sounds like a cliché, if she really likes you, the fact that you have psoriasis will not make a difference to how she feels. In terms of how you tell her, you can take one of two approaches. You can tell her straight out yourself or, if you find this too difficult, you could tell her that you have psoriasis and give her some information leaflets to read up about it herself. In general, people tend to find that they feel much better once they have told their girlfriend/boyfriend, as there is then nothing to hide.

What can I do to avoid embarrassment in personal relationships?

The best way to avoid embarrassment is to be as up-front as possible with your partner. By explaining what psoriasis is, you help to get round some of the awkward feelings. As we have said before, psoriasis is not your fault and does not reflect badly on you as a person. Trying to keep this in mind when you approach your personal relationships may help you to avoid embarrassment.

I have psoriasis on my penis and find it quite painful to have sex. What is the best treatment to use?

Because the skin on your penis is relatively delicate, this limits the range of treatments you can use on it. The preferred treatment is usually a mild topical steroid – using a moisturiser may help to soothe it and lessen any scaling. Using condoms may help protect your penis and make sex less painful. Do be aware that most condoms are damaged by oil-based substances (e.g. baby oil) and any ointments. If these substances are on your penis, the condom will not be safe. Durex, however, have made a type of condom called Avanti which they claim is safe for use with oil-based substances, so you should be safe with this type of condom after using ointments.

If for some reason you don't use condoms, applying a lubricant when having sex might make it less uncomfortable. Do not have sexual intercourse after applying any of the active treatments to your penis; they are not intended for internal use and might affect your partner badly. The other thing to bear in mind is that the friction your penis experiences during sex may aggravate the psoriasis. Refraining from having sexual intercourse until the psoriasis goes may be an option you and your partner could consider. Of course, in the meantime, there are other ways of expressing loving feelings – for example, cuddling and fondling.

My wife is very hard to live with since she developed psoriasis. Can it affect a person's character?

Living with psoriasis is very distressing for some people and may, as a consequence, change the way they behave. Not only can psoriasis give a great deal of physical discomfort, it can also affect a person's self-esteem and the way they feel about themselves. These two things together may seem to change a person's character. We suggest that you try to talk to your wife about how she feels – she may think that you feel differently towards her now that she has psoriasis, and you need to reassure her. In a very practical sense, it is important that she gets the best treatment available; a visit to the doctor or practice nurse may be helpful to ensure that her treatment is as good as possible. Your GP might be able to refer her to a psychologist, which some people find very helpful.

Finally, talking to others with psoriasis is a good way of getting support and makes people realise they are not alone. The Psoriasis Association has local groups that do a lot of good work, fund raising and increasing the profile of psoriasis in society. Your local group can be contacted through the national association (address in Appendix 1). If there isn't one nearby, perhaps you and your wife could start the ball rolling? Although the main focus of the Psoriatic Arthropathy Alliance (address in Appendix 1) is for people with psoriatic arthropathy, they also provide information about psoriasis. Some dermatology departments offer specific support groups and it is worth contacting your local hospital to see if such a service exists.

My 25-year-old son has just developed psoriasis and I feel so guilty about this that I can't talk to him about it. What should I do?

First of all, the guilt you are experiencing is quite commonly felt by parents when their children develop psoriasis. Although your feelings are understandable, there is no point in your blaming yourself, because it is not something that you can have had any control over. Whilst the susceptibility for psoriasis is inherited, many people carry this gene unknowingly as they do not develop the active symptoms themselves. What is most important is that you do talk to your son about it. One of the things that makes coping with psoriasis easier is to have people around you who support and help you. At this potentially difficult time of his life, your son will need your understanding more than ever. If you approach him and he does not want to talk about it, it is probably best to respect this, but make sure that he knows that if he *does* want to talk you will always be there for him.

Feeling 'different'

I feel so isolated and alone – nobody seems to understand what's happened to me.

Many people with psoriasis feel isolated and alone with their condition. The statistics, however, tell a different story: at least 1 in every 50 people has psoriasis – think how many people at your average football match must have it! Isolation often occurs because people feel unable to talk to others about their psoriasis, especially when it has first been diagnosed. The most effective way of getting round the feelings of isolation is to seek support from others around you. Although you may feel embarrassed to talk about psoriasis, others will not be able to help or support you unless you do and thus let them know how you are feeling. Support groups are good places to find help: the people there understand what you are going through, as it is likely that they will have had similar experiences themselves. Addresses of possible support groups are given in Appendix 1.

My psoriasis is ruining my life. Everything I try to do seems to be affected by the state of my skin and I can't look forward to anything. How can I change this?

Your story is only too familiar. Psoriasis can rule your life. To break free and change the way it affects you, you may need the help of a psychologist, and your GP or consultant should be able to refer you to one. People often cope with psoriasis by avoiding situations that might cause embarrassment from other people's comments. Examples include not accepting invitations to stay with family or friends for fear of leaving scales on the floor, and not exposing your skin to the sun even though it would probably help. A psychologist will work with you to change the way you feel about yourself and your skin.

Psychologists cannot change the fact that you have psoriasis but they can influence the way you think about it. As well as this they teach relaxation techniques, and interpersonal and social skills. You should end up feeling much more confident in yourself as a person, with a degree of control over your psoriasis so that it no longer dominates your life.

I get so irate when people say to me 'it's only skin', as if having psoriasis is not a serious problem.

It is true that many members of the public do not understand the serious impact that psoriasis can have on people's lives. Because psoriasis is rarely life threatening and the skin is seen as not that important, they do not appreciate the severe physical and psychological discomfort that it can cause. What you can do in these situations is try to explain how it feels to you having psoriasis and also point out how important the skin is as an organ of the body. For example, the skin is the largest organ of the body, and is responsible for protection, temperature regulation, sensing pleasure and pain, defence mechanisms through the immune system and, of course, our appearance. All you need to do is look at the beauty industry to see how important the appearance of the skin is!

The next time someone makes an insensitive comment about it 'only being skin', you be ready with your response so that they are left in no doubt about the important role the skin has to play in health and well-being!

I feel like it is all my fault that I have got psoriasis and blame myself for letting it wreck my life.

It is quite common that people blame themselves for having psoriasis, but let us look at the facts. There is no doubt that to have psoriasis you need to have the gene or genes that make you susceptible to it. You could not have done anything about this. To show active signs of psoriasis, this gene needs to be activated or triggered. These trigger factors have been discussed in Chapter 3. Most people at some point in life experience one or more of these trigger factors, and they will respond to them in different ways. For you, your body responds by developing psoriasis; this is not your fault and you should not blame yourself for it. The aim of this book and of the various support groups that exist is to help people to make sure that having psoriasis does not wreck their lives. The hope is that, by highlighting ways of managing it both physically and psychologically, people will feel better able to live life to the full and make the most of it.

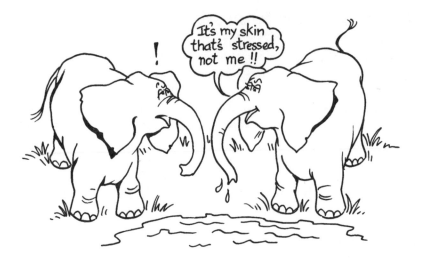

A lot of people say that stress is what causes psoriasis. I always feel as if they are suggesting that I don't cope well with stress when in fact I think I am quite a calm and 'together' person. What do you think?

There is little doubt that stress is one of the potential trigger factors for psoriasis. However, the point you are making is one commonly reflected by others with psoriasis – they get fed up with people saying it is stress that causes psoriasis and insinuating that the individual must be unable to cope with the stress in their life or else they wouldn't have developed the condition. Although the evidence does point to stress having an effect on the development of psoriasis, this does not automatically mean that you are bad at coping with it. We all experience difficult situations in our lives, and, although the experience of stress is affected by our psychological state, it is also a physiological response that happens automatically in our bodies and over which we have little control. As with most things in psoriasis, this is very individual: some people are absolutely certain that experiencing stress makes their psoriasis worse; others do not see such a direct link. Lumping everyone together and making generalisations is not helpful and not especially accurate.

Feeling embarrassed

I get so embarrassed when I go out because I can't help scratching.

Psoriasis can be very itchy indeed and it is difficult to stop yourself scratching – people often find that they do it subconsciously without even noticing. Because of this it is helpful to keep your finger nails short so that, if you *do* scratch, you cause less damage. Once you start scratching, although you might get relief at first, it often makes you feel itchier in the long run. Stopping scratching can therefore make you feel less itchy.

Your skin is less likely to be itchy if your treatment is effective. Moisturising, in particular, is very helpful because it is cooling and soothing, and you can apply lots of it. Rather than scratching, try applying some moisturiser. The principles of moisturising apply to your scalp as well as to your body – massaging coconut oil into the scalp acts as an excellent moisturiser.

Other helpful tips to minimise the likelihood of your scratching while you are out include wearing cool, loose-fitting cotton clothing and avoiding sitting close to direct sources of heat. If you can be aware of what your hands are doing (e.g. folding them on the table), this can reduce the temptation to scratch. Some people use a 'counter' that they click each time they want to scratch; this just increases your awareness of the desire to scratch and can decrease your scratching dramatically. Finally, if you are with close friends or family, it might be worth asking them to tell you when you are scratching so you can stop before you really get going.

I sometimes get a bit of psoriasis on my face and I am very aware of people looking at it when I am talking to them rather than focusing on what I am saying. What can I do?

People will always look at blemishes on someone's face – one's eyes are so often drawn towards a spot or a patch of psoriasis. It is quite unnerving, though, when you are trying to get a serious message across, to feel that they are not concentrating on what you are saying. Really the only solution, other than ploughing on regardless of the stares, is to try to make the patch of psoriasis less obvious by applying lots of moisturiser and by using a cover-up make-up. This last suggestion is easier for women to follow, but the British Red Cross and the British Association of Skin Camouflage (addresses in Appendix 1) offer a very effective camouflage service using special techniques to cover up unwanted skin changes.

If you know the person you are speaking to, you may feel comfortable enough to tell them that you have psoriasis and mention that they seem to be staring. This tactic is harder if you are talking to a stranger but why not try it – you might be pleasantly surprised by their response.

Feeling fed up

The treatments that I have been given to do are so time consuming and expensive that I feel like just giving up and living with the psoriasis.

This is a decision that you are of course free to take. It is your skin and if you feel able to cope with it not using any treatment then that is absolutely fine. However, before you take this decision, it is probably worth considering three points. First, have you and your doctor explored all the possible options for treatment – are you perhaps just fed up because you don't have a treatment that fits in with your life-style? Secondly, have you explored all the options for getting cheaper prescriptions (see Chapter 10) if cost is a real problem? And, thirdly, if you stop doing anything, your psoriasis may get worse.

If you do decide to stop treating your skin with any active treatments, it would be very wise to continue moisturising. Choose a nice light lotion, which can be very quick to apply and will have a minimal impact on your life but will help to keep the psoriasis less dry and therefore more comfortable.

My doctor is too busy with people who have problems more serious than mine to keep bothering her about different treatments.

It might sometimes seem this way, but it is important that you feel able to see your GP whenever you need to to discuss the treatments you are using and whether they are working or not. Your GP is there to provide care to *all* the patients on her books and she will not think that you are any less important than the other people she sees. If, however, you feel that you are not getting the information you need about the treatments from your GP, you might like to ask whether there is anyone else who can help – there may be a nurse available who has more time to discuss things with you. It may also be worth considering making contact with the Psoriatic Arthropathy Alliance or the Psoriasis Association. Both are organisations with access to information about treatments as well as being support groups of people with psoriasis who may be experiencing the same sort of thing as you.

9
Life-style and looks

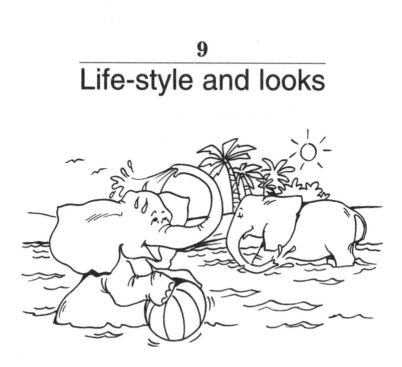

Introduction

Any glance at a magazine rack in a shop will show the number of publications for men and women dealing with life-style and looks. In this chapter we hope to provide answers that can help you to avoid problems in achieving the look you want and in living life in the way you want. This is not always easy. People with psoriasis are well known for buying patterned carpets because these help to disguise the shed scales!

These days, many diseases are judged by the impact they have on quality of life, and studies have shown that psoriasis is up there with heart disease over the problems it can cause. In one study, people unlucky enough to have both diabetes and psoriasis were more likely to choose psoriasis if offered the imaginary chance of a cure for one of their diseases. All health care workers should ask patients with psoriasis about the impact of the disease on areas such as holidays, work, sport and their sex-life. People often won't bother the doctor with what they consider are trivial questions but they are probably the most important issues to deal with if life with psoriasis is to be as normal as possible.

Clothes

What are the best types of clothes/material to wear?

The short answer is 'Whatever feels most comfortable to you'. Smooth fabrics that do not rub or aggravate plaques are probably the best (e.g. soft cotton or silk). Sometimes creases or seams can be uncomfortable if they rub psoriasis and are best avoided – likewise, tight trousers might worsen plaques on your legs.

If you are applying very messy, greasy treatments, you will find it easier to have a set of clothes (e.g. shirt and track suit) that you put on while the treatment sinks in.

My psoriasis seems to be worse where my clothes rub, for example round my waist. Why is this?

'Koebner's phenomenon' is the medical term for what you have described. Psoriasis can get worse in areas where skin is rubbed or damaged in any way. So, for example, where you fall over and cut yourself, psoriasis is more likely to form in the scar; or if you have an operation, psoriasis is more likely to form along the line where the surgical cut was made. Also, if you constantly scratch or pick your psoriasis, this is also likely to make it worse. Note that there is not a 100% link – psoriasis will not always form at the point of injury – but it significantly increases the likelihood. The skin does not have to be broken to cause Koebner's phenomenon, as this question demonstrates; it can occur where constant rubbing is present.

My washing machine gets ruined by all the grease that I have to use as part of my treatments. Can you make any suggestion as to how to prolong the life of my machine?

The grease in the heavier duty moisturisers (the ointments) causes the rubber seal around the washing machine door to disintegrate. There is, as yet, no total solution to this but Hotpoint suggest that the rubber seals can be made to last longer by periodically doing an empty wash at 35 degrees Celsius (95 degrees Fahrenheit) with biological powder. (This presumably dissolves the grease and makes it less likely to damage the rubber.) Writing to washing machine manufacturers about this problem will ensure that they know it is a real problem for users – and hopefully encourage them to develop more durable rubber seals!

There are a couple of other practical measures you can take that might help to prolong the life of your machine. First, if you have garments that are heavily impregnated with grease, soak them in a bowl of very hot water with some washing detergent or, perhaps better, soda crystals – this will help to remove some of the grease. The second possibility is to change your moisturiser to one that is less greasy. This will obviously depend on how severe your psoriasis is, but it may be possible to use a less greasy moisturiser more often and still keep your skin adequately moisturised. If it is the active treatment that is making your garments greasy, you might consider asking your doctor to prescribe you the cream rather than the ointment form. Although creams tend to be less good than ointments at keeping your skin moisturised, they are more acceptable cosmetically.

Staining

Clothes and soft furnishing get very stained with the treatments. Can you suggest ways of preventing this or of removing the marks?

Once soft furnishings are stained, it is generally difficult to remove the stains. If it is possible to hot wash them, this may get rid of grease stains but tar and Dithrocream tend to stay put. If you get tar or Dithrocream on the floor or furniture, remove it with a cloth as quickly as possible (this limits the staining).

The best course of action, therefore, is prevention and, failing that, 'damage limitation'. If you are using tar or Dithrocream at home, make sure you have some sets of clothes that you wear after the treatment; this way you ruin only a limited number of garments. Try always to do your treatment in one place – probably the bathroom – and stand on old towels to protect the flooring. When you have finished doing the treatment, use old towels to protect furnishings. If you are doing a scalp treatment, try to do it before bed and go to bed with the treatment on, protecting your pillows with two or three old pillowcases.

Another possible course of action is to ask your doctor whether you could change to a less messy treatment option; this may not always be appropriate, though. You might also like to ask for some tubular cotton bandages (e.g. Tubifast), which can be used to help keep the treatment in place and stop it getting rubbed off.

Cosmetics and personal appearance

Can I wear make-up when I have got psoriasis?

There is no reason why you cannot wear make-up. If you have psoriasis on your face, which you want to cover up with make-up, do a small test area first to make sure that the make-up does not aggravate it. Be sure to remove make-up at the end of the day and then apply plenty of moisturiser.

My 12-year-old wants to get her ears pierced. Will this make her psoriasis worse?

If she is careful and uses an experienced piercer rather than doing it herself or letting a friend do it, she should have no problems. There are some risks, however. She might develop psoriasis at the site of piercing (Koebner's phenomenon) or, if she

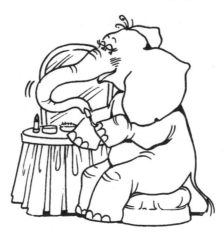

developed an infection, this might cause a general flare-up. Having her ears pierced is part of being normal despite the psoriasis, so we would suggest that you allow her to go ahead.

Can I wear nail polish?

Yes, nail polish is fine for you to use. Be a bit careful with nail polish remover because, if you have sore fingertips, this will make them sting.

Will dyeing my hair do the psoriasis in my scalp any harm?

When considering dyeing your hair the thing to be careful about is worsening the scalp psoriasis by applying astringent chemicals to it. Bleaching hair, for example, would probably make scalp psoriasis worse. Hair dyes are much less aggressive than they used to be and you may well be able to find one that suits. However, our advice is that you do not try tinting or colouring your hair at home but that you take advice from your hairdresser, who should have the most up-to-date information about possible options. Hairdressers are taught about skin conditions that affect the scalp and should be knowledgeable enough to offer advice.

Many people feel embarrassed about going to the hairdressers, but a good hairdresser will not shy away from doing your hair. If you feel concerned about going to the hairdressers, why not try phoning first and explaining your situation to one of the stylists?

If they sound sympathetic over the phone, you can book to see them and you won't have to feel you need to do any explaining once you are there.

Quite large lumps of my hair have come out. Is this normal?

It is quite usual for hair to fall out when psoriasis is active in your scalp. When you descale your scalp, you may find that your hair seems to fall out more particularly – especially when the plaques are treated or when you comb or brush it. Although it is worrying to see your hair come out, it will grow back once the scalp psoriasis has been successfully treated.

Can I remove hair from my legs?

Yes, you can. But if you shave and cut yourself, this might lead to new patches of psoriasis appearing (Koebner's phenomenon, discussed earlier). Also note that plaques of psoriasis tend to bleed more easily than other skin and therefore waxing or sugaring your legs might cause pinprick bleeding (i.e. little specks of blood across the surface of the plaque).

Applying treatments seems to make the psoriasis look worse. Is this true and, if so, why?

This does seem to be the case for many people. Applying ointments or creams to your skin gets rid of the scaliness on top of the plaques, which then emphasises the redness of the plaque underneath. This seems to be the case particularly if a greasy ointment is used. If you are rubbing the ointments into the plaques, this can cause the blood vessels to dilate so that the blood comes to the surface of the skin, thus increasing the red appearance.

There are two things you can do to minimise the impact that this has on you. First of all, if you find that the treatment makes your psoriasis look redder, try to apply it with sufficient time for the redness to die down before you go out. Secondly, apply the treatment gently (although you do need to rub it in). Don't, whatever you do, stop the treatments: although they might make the plaque look worse temporarily, they are doing a good job and will show good results in the long run.

I have quite dark skin and I find that after I clear the plaques of psoriasis I am left with patches of lighter skin. Is there anything I can do about this?

It does seem that, on clearing the psoriasis, people are sometimes left with areas of skin that are lighter than the rest of the skin; this will be particularly obvious if you have dark skin. These areas will eventually 'recover' and the normal pigmentation will return – but it may take up to a year. This phenomenon occurs in all skin types but is more noticeable in dark or tanned skin.

Swimming

Will it hurt or worsen if I go swimming?

No – swimming itself does not harm your psoriasis. If you swim in a chlorinated swimming pool (as opposed to the sea or a lake), the chlorine can have a drying effect on your skin. Making sure that you wash your skin very thoroughly following your swim and applying plenty of moisturiser before you get dressed can counterbalance this.

You may find that some people will stare or make unpleasant comments when you go swimming, but most will probably take very little notice. You should not be asked to leave the pool by the authorities but you might feel more comfortable approaching the pool manager before getting into the pool, just to check that they are not going to object. It is important to tell people that psoriasis is not catching; sometimes they can be ignorant about what psoriasis is, which makes them react in a negative way. It could be worth taking some information literature with you to give to anyone who asks you, which will save you having to explain yourself. You can photocopy Appendix 4, which has the basic facts for you to pass on.

Some support groups arrange special sessions at a pool, so that there is more than one person with psoriasis there, or a session specifically for people with psoriasis. In any case, try to be confident: remember that you have as much right to swim and enjoy yourself as any one else.

I'd rather die than feel noticeable. What can I do to avoid embarrassment on the beach or in the swimming pool?

Often the embarrassment is caused by wondering what other people are thinking about your psoriasis. There are two ways of coping with this. First, ignore the odd glance that you may get – generally people are a lot less interested than you think they are. We are all 'guilty' of looking at people around us to see what they are wearing, how they look in a swimsuit etc. – it is no more than a passing interest. Secondly, confront people in a polite but firm way, especially if you feel they really are staring at you. Have ready prepared in your head a little spiel that you come out with – for example, 'I have a skin condition called psoriasis. It is quite common. It makes my skin grow too fast . . . and don't worry, because you can't catch it.' Most people will accept this sort of explanation.

As mentioned in the answer above, you have as much right as anyone else to swim or lie on the beach. It is not your fault that you have psoriasis and it doesn't make you any less of a good person. The embarrassment is something you feel in yourself – use the support of your friends and family to help you get over it. Take them with you when you go swimming so that you don't feel so vulnerable or isolated. Most of all, enjoy yourself and try not to focus on what you think other people are thinking about you.

Other considerations

Should I give up smoking?

Yes, you should give up smoking – the health benefits of doing so are significant for everyone. Some research suggests that smokers are twice as likely as non-smokers to develop psoriasis. Smoking is bad for your skin in general, as it speeds up the ageing process. So, although stopping smoking will probably not make your psoriasis go away, it might help contribute to it not coming back again and it will certainly have a very positive effect on your overall health as well as on the quality of your skin.

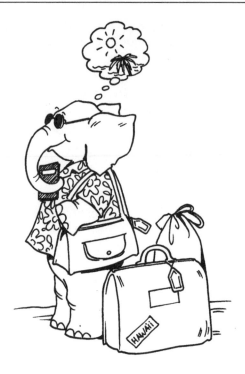

Would it help if I emigrated?

There is little doubt that sunny weather helps control psoriasis for many people, so, for them, living in a sunny climate might well help. However, sunshine is not helpful for everyone, and for some it worsens their condition. If you were to seriously think about emigrating, you should also give consideration to the health services available in the country you hope to go to. In some countries (e.g. South Africa, New Zealand and the USA), you might not have access to a public health service, so the cost of private health care needs to be carefully considered.

Would it help if I lost weight?

If you are definitely overweight, losing weight will not do you any harm and indeed will significantly benefit your overall health and well-being. It is unlikely, however, to have a direct effect on your psoriasis. Having said this, being overweight can give you extra folds of fat, which produce deep creases in which you can develop psoriasis. These areas can be difficult to treat, so losing weight can make life easier in terms of being able to do treatments. If the fact that you are overweight gives you concern and makes you feel less good about yourself, resolving this might help to put you in a better frame of mind to cope with and manage your psoriasis.

If I had a large patch of psoriasis taken off and a skin graft done, would it stay away forever?

No, it would not stay away. Psoriasis develops because of changes occurring in the immune system. These changes would affect a new skin graft in the same way that they affect your old skin.

10

Practical concerns

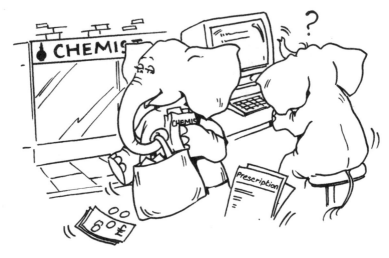

Introduction

In this chapter we try to answer the many questions that people ask about the financial and other practical aspects of living with psoriasis, including what is happening in medical research.

Money questions

Is there any way of reducing the cost of prescription charges if I have to have several items a month?

Yes. If you are one of the minority in this country who pay for prescriptions, you can lessen the burden by obtaining a prepayment certificate. Your GP or pharmacist should have details about how to obtain this from your local health authority, using form FP95 (EP95 in Scotland). The price is linked to the cost of prescriptions, so it can change when prescription charges are altered, but if you have more than five items in three months or more than 14 in a year it is well worth doing. Certificates can cover a quarter or a full year.

It is also worth checking whether you are exempt from prescription charges for any other reason. You can get a leaflet entitled *Are you entitled to help with health cost?* available from post offices, Social Security offices or hospitals. In general, people who do not have to pay for prescriptions are:

* people aged 60 or over,
* people aged under 16,
* people aged 16, 17 and 18 who are in full-time education,
* people (and their adult dependants) receiving Income Support, income-based JobSeekers' Allowance, Family Credit or Disabled Person's Tax Credit (formerly Disability Working Allowance),
* women who are pregnant or have a baby under 12 months old,
* people with certain medical conditions (psoriasis is *not* one of them),
* people who receive a War or Ministry of Defence Disablement Pension who need prescriptions because of their disability.

Note This list is correct at the time of writing but you can be sure with such lists that the contents will vary. Consult your GP or pharmacy or the local Citizens Advice Bureau for the latest information.

Some of the treatments that are used for psoriasis are available over the counter (without a prescription). Buying them this way is sometimes cheaper than getting a prescription. However, do note that sometimes it works the other way, something obtained with a prescription being cheaper than buying it over the counter.

The Tables in Appendix 3 will give you some idea of comparative costs, although clearly prices do change.

My husband has very bad psoriasis and the arthritis that goes with it. I am unable to work as I have to care for him, and we have very little money. Are there any benefits we could claim?

Yes, at least two come to mind. Your husband could be eligible for Disability Living Allowance (DLA). This is not means-tested so any savings or other income he has will not affect it. DLA is based on the amount of care needed and varies depending on day and night needs. It also has a component for mobility and this can lead into special interest-free loans for a car. You could also avoid having to pay the road fund licence; this is covered under the Motability scheme (address in Appendix 1).

If your husband gets DLA, you may be entitled to claim Invalid Care Allowance for yourself. You would have to be spending 35 hours or more a week caring for him. This benefit is also not means-tested but does have to be declared for tax purposes. Further information is available from any Benefits Agency office or from the Benefit Enquiry Line on 0800 88 22 00. Leaflet N1196 covers all the Social Security Benefit rates.

Jobs

Are there any jobs that I cannot apply for because I have got psoriasis?

You can apply for any job that you want – the response you receive to your application will depend largely on the current state of your psoriasis and how bad it has been in the past. Many employers will have very little interest in the fact that you have psoriasis, particularly if it has not had an adverse effect on your previous employment record. However, there are some employers – including the armed forces – who are more likely to question you about your psoriasis and perhaps even reject you because of it. It is important to note that this is not a blanket approach and their ideas are often out of date; if you have a real passion for doing a specific job, you should apply for it on the assumption that individual assessments need to be made.

On a personal level, it is important for you to think through the impact of your psoriasis on any job you might do. If, for example, you have very bad psoriasis on your hands and/or under your finger nails, this might make doing a job that involves fine movements with your fingers difficult and painful. If you are the right person for a job, a good employer should help you to find ways of coping with your psoriasis at work so that it has a minimum impact on your comfort and what you do. Occupational health departments in the workplace are often helpful sources of information and support. JobCentres have disability advisers who may be able to provide information about jobs and benefits that you might be eligible for.

The future

What hopes are there for a cure in the future?

A cure for psoriasis may be possible at some point in the future. However, it is unlikely to happen in the next few years. Current research suggests that there is more than one gene linked to psoriasis – possibly as many as six – which in turn suggests that there are a number of different types of psoriasis. Research on this issue may lead to the development of new treatments that are better targeted to the specific type of psoriasis. Thus in the future it is likely that increasingly effective treatments will be developed, which will make managing the disease less of a problem and make life easier.

Is there much research being done?

There is research going on in a number of different areas:

* Genetic research to identify the gene (or genes) that causes (or cause) people to develop psoriasis.
* Exploration of the immune system – especially T-lymphocytes (a type of white cell), which are thought to have a major contributory effect on the development of psoriasis. Manipulation of the immune system may eventually provide us with some 'cures' for psoriasis.

- Looking for different and better treatments for psoriasis means developing new creams, ointments and tablets.
- The effect that psoriasis has on people's lives. The information gained helps health care professionals have a better understanding of its impact and helps to improve dermatology services. This research is also used to improve public awareness and understanding of psoriasis.

There are many different institutions and organisations undertaking research. They often need volunteers to take part in the research. If you want to find out about being a volunteer, patients' organisations often have information about current research projects.

More help and information

My GP does not seem to know or care. How can I get to see a specialist?

There are two ways that you can get to see a skin specialist (dermatologist): either through your GP or by paying to see one privately. If your GP refuses to refer you to a dermatologist, you could ask to talk to another GP to see if they are of the same opinion, but it is definitely worth discussing with your GP why he or she does not think you need referral to a specialist.

You are, of course, free to change GPs if you want to, and you could look for one who has a special interest in, and therefore more knowledge of, dermatology. If you decide that you want to see someone privately, you may be able to do this yourself by contacting a dermatologist directly. More often than not, though, you will still need a letter from your GP referring you to a specialist even if you go privately. Make sure that you know how much it is going to cost before you make a private appointment.

My GP says I do not need to go to hospital but I think I do, and I don't like using the steroids he gives me.

It is quite difficult if you fundamentally disagree with your GP about the care he is offering you. The best way to tackle this is to be prepared next time you go to see him. Take a list of questions asking why he is prescribing the treatment he is and requesting a trial of something else. Topical steroids are sometimes helpful for some types of psoriasis, but they are not generally considered to be the best long-term treatment, so you are right to think about asking for an alternative. If you feel you need hospital treatment, you should ask your GP to explain why he believes that hospital treatment is inappropriate. You can ask to talk to another GP in the practice to see if he or she has an alternative opinion.

I sometimes feel so confused about how to apply my treatments. I know my GP is too busy to spend much time explaining these to me. Is there anyone else who might be able to help?

It is quite understandable that you might feel a bit confused about which treatments to use when and how to apply them. This sort of support is what specialist nurses who have a specific interest in skin disease can offer. Some GP practices are now looking at the possibility of employing a nurse with this sort of expertise so that they can improve the care offered to people with skin disease, including psoriasis. This idea is in the early stages of being tried out but it may well spread to more and more practices, so it is worth checking with your GP to see if they have such a service in mind.

I have noticed that a high street chemists shop has started to offer skin care advice through 'skin care advisers'. What do you think about this?

It is not the place of this book to comment on the quality of the advice offered by these advisers, but we believe that you should make sure that you know what you will get if you consult one of them. You should ask questions for the following reasons:

• They are not members of a professional body, so members of the public are not protected through the usual mechanisms offered by professions such as nursing, medicine and pharmacy.
• Although they will have received some in-house training, this will not have been approved by any statutory or professional

bodies, so the standard will not have been guaranteed by an impartial organisation.

• Because they are employed by a commercial organisation, they are likely to be promoting products made by that organisation or at least advocating the use of products sold in that shop. These products may not necessarily be the ones that are best for you.

On a positive note, it is encouraging that a major chemists chain is recognising the impact that skin problems have and providing an advisory service that it hopes will do something to help. It is important, however, that the public be aware that the advice may well not be impartial.

How can I find out about the most recent treatments available?

Your GP will have some information about recent treatments, but is unlikely to be aware of everything that is available. The Psoriasis Association is a very good source of information and its newsletter (distributed to all members three times a year) often contains reviews about new treatments on the market. Your local hospital dermatology department is likely to have information about latest treatments, but it is not always easy to get at this information unless you have an appointment with the department. If you have access to the Internet, the British Association of Dermatologists' website (address in Appendix 1) provides a lot of information. The Psoriatic Arthropathy Alliance offers excellent information through newsletters and a journal, as well as a CD-ROM. It also holds an annual conference, which has useful presentations, exhibits, discussions and so on.

Where can I get more information about psoriasis?

Appendix 1 of this book includes organisations and sources of information that you can use to find out more. There are increasing numbers of addresses available on the Internet. Putting the word 'psoriasis' into a search 'engine' will find a number of these, but in Appendix 1 are some that we have checked out.

Glossary

Terms in *italic* in the definitions below are also defined in this Glossary.

acute   Short-lasting. In medical terms, this usually means lasting for days rather than weeks or months. (*See also* chronic)

adrenal glands   Important glands in the body that produce a number of *hormones* to control the body systems. Cortisol and cortisone are two very important examples, and adrenaline is another.

allergy   To have an allergy means to over-react to something in a harmful way when you come into contact with it. If you have an allergy to grass pollen, you will have streaming eyes and nose and sneezing if you come into contact with it (hayfever). Someone who is not allergic to grass pollen will not even notice when they have come into contact with it.

anaemia   This means a reduction in the amount of the oxygen-carrying pigment, haemoglobin, in the blood.

anecdotal evidence   Reports from people about their experience of *triggers*, treatments etc. – rather than scientific evidence obtained from strictly regulated tests.

antibody   A special kind of blood protein made in response to a particular *antigen*, which is designed to attack the antigen.

antigen   Any substance that the body regards as foreign or potentially dangerous.

arthritis   Inflammation of one or more joints, characterised by swelling, heat, redness of overlying skin, pain and restriction of movement.

atrophy   Wasting away of a body tissue. With skin this means thinning and loss of strength.

barrier cream A cream or ointment used to protect the skin against irritants.

biopsy The process of obtaining a sample of tissue (e.g. liver or skin) for analysis under a microscope.

bone marrow The tissue contained in the internal cavities of bones that is involved in making blood cells.

chronic In strictly medical terms, chronic means long-lasting or persistent. Many people use the word 'chronic' incorrectly to mean severe or extreme. (*See also* acute)

cytotoxic Something that can damage cells.

dermatology The medical speciality concerned with the diagnosis and treatment of skin disease.

dermis The deep layer of the skin.

diagnostic Something that is 'diagnostic' is a characteristic feature; it occurs so often in a disease that you don't need any other clues to know what the disease is.

distribution The pattern of a disease on the skin; for example, all over, on the hands, in the *flexures*, etc.

eczema A red, itchy inflammation of the skin, sometimes with blisters and weeping.

emollient An agent that soothes and softens the skin; also known as a moisturiser.

emulsifying ointment A thick, greasy *emollient*.

epidermis The outer layer of the skin.

erythroderma An abnormal reddening, flaking and thickening of the skin, affecting a wide area of the body.

extensor The side of a limb on which lie the muscles that straighten the limb (e.g. the back of the arm and the front of the leg).

flexures The areas where the limbs bend, bringing two skin surfaces close together (e.g. the creases at the front of the elbows, the back of the knees and the groin).

genes 'Units' of inheritance that make up an individual's characteristics. Half are inherited from each parent.

genetic To do with *genes*.

guttate A term used to describe lesions on the skin that are shaped like drops of water

hormone A substance that is produced in a gland in one part of the body and is carried in the bloodstream to work in other parts of the body.

immune system The body's defence system against outside 'attackers' whether they are infections, injuries or agents that are recognised as 'foreign' (e.g. a transplanted organ). The immune system fights off infection and produces *antibodies* that will protect against future attack.

immunity Resistance to specific disease(s) because of *antibodies* produced by the body's *immune system*.

immuno-suppressive A drug that reduces the body's resistance to infection and other foreign bodies by suppressing the immune reaction.

in-patient therapy Treatment carried out when a patient is admitted to hospital.

incidence The number of new cases of an illness arising in a population over a given time.

inflammation The reaction of the body to an injury, infection or disease. Generally, it will protect the body against the spread of injury or infection, but may become *chronic*, when it tends to damage the body rather than protect it.

interleukin-2 One of a group of special proteins that control the immune response. Interleukin-2 stimulates the T-*lymphocytes* that are active in the skin.

keratinocytes Types of cells that make up over 95% of the *epidermis* (outer layer of the skin).

Koebner's phenomenon This describes a reaction in the skin that occurs in psoriasis and some other skin diseases, where typical lesions of the disease appear in areas of skin damaged by injury such as a scratch, cut or burn.

liver biopsy *See* biopsy

lymphocytes White blood cells that are involved in *immunity*.

malnutrition The condition resulting from an improper balance between what is eaten and what the body needs.

moisturiser *See* emollient.

natural history The normal course of a disease, the way it develops over time.

non-steroidal anti-inflammatory drugs (NSAIDs) A group of drugs that act to reduce inflammation in the body, particularly in rheumatic diseases.

papular A pattern of rash that consists of small raised spots on the skin less than 5mm across.

photosensitiser Any agent, *topical* or *systemic*, that acts to increase the sensitivity of the skin to light.

phototherapy Treatment with light – usually ultra-violet (UV) light.

placebo A medicine that is ineffective but may help to relieve a condition because the patient has faith in its powers. New drugs are tested against placebos to make sure that they have a true active benefit in addition to the 'placebo response'.

plaque   A raised patch on the skin more than 2cm across.

psoriasis   A *chronic* inflammatory skin disease.

psychologist   A specialist who studies behaviour and its related mental processes.

pustules   A small pus-containing blister.

sebaceous glands   Glands in the skin that produce an oily substance – sebum.

seborrhoeic   Related to excessive secretion of sebum (*see also* sebaceous glands).

seborrhoeic eczema   A form of eczema that affects the face, scalp, upper back and chest. It characteristically produces yellowish greasy scales.

spondylo-arthritis   A term used to describe arthritis of the spine.

steroids   A particular group of chemicals, which includes very important *hormones*, produced naturally by the body, and also many drugs used for a wide range of medical purposes. In psoriasis the subgroup of steroids with which we are concerned is the corticosteroids. Very often this term is shortened to 'steroids', causing people to confuse their skin treatments with the anabolic steroids used for body building.

subcutaneous   Beneath the skin.

systemic   This term is used for a drug, given by mouth or injection, that affects the whole body.

teratogenic   Something that damages an unborn child.

topical   A term used to describe drugs that are applied to the skin rather than being taken internally.

triggers   Factors that may bring on psoriasis but do not cause psoriasis.

Appendix 1

Useful addresses

Please note that website addresses change quite frequently and quickly become out of date.

Patient support organisations

Psoriasis Association
Milton House
7 Milton Street
Northampton NN2 7JG
Tel: 01604 711129
Fax: 01604 792894
Offers useful information and support about various aspects of psoriasis.

Psoriatic Arthropathy Alliance
PO Box 111
St Albans
Hertfordshire AL2 3JQ
Tel: 01923 682606
Fax: 01923 672837
Email: info@paalliance.org
Website: www.paalliance.org
Offers useful information and support about various aspects of psoriasis.

Skin Care Campaign
163 Eversholt Street
London NW1 1BU
Tel: 020 7388 4097
Fax: 020 7388 5882
An alliance of patient groups, health professionals and other organisations concerned with skin care. It campaigns for a better deal for people with a wide variety of skin problems.

Skinship
10 Thurstable Way
Tollesbury
Maldon
Essex CM9 8SQ
Tel: 01621 868666
Fax: 01621 363001
*Provides a helpline for people
with any skin disease, the aim
being to 'ease the pain and end
the shame'.*

Other useful sources of information

All Party Parliamentary Group on
Skin (now the Associate
Parliamentary Group on Skin)
3/19 Holmbush Road
London SW15 3LE
Tel: 020 8789 2798
Fax: 020 8789 0795
*An all-party group specialising
in skin, which was established
in 1993 to raise awareness in
Parliament of skin disease.*

Association of the British
Pharmaceutical Industry
12 Whitehall
London SW1A 2DY
Tel: 020 7930 3477
Fax: 020 7747 1411
Email: abpi@abpi.org.uk
*Brings together companies in
Britain producing prescription
medicines, other organisations
involved in pharmaceutical
research and development, and
those with an interest in the
pharmaceutical industry in the
UK.*

Benefits Agency
*For advice about state benefits.
Leaflet N1196 covers all the
Social Security benefit rates. See
the telephone directory for your
local Benefits Agency office.*

Benefits Enquiry Line
Tel: 0800 88 22 00
Website: www/dss/gov/uk/ba
*State benefits information line
for sick or disabled people and
their carers.*

British Association of
Dermatologists/British
Dermatological Nursing Group
19 Fitzroy Square
London W1P 5HQ
Tel: 020 7383 0266
Fax: 020 7388 5263
Email: admin@bad.org.uk
Website: www.bad.org.uk
*Professional organisations
representing doctors and nurses
who have an interest in and/or
work directly in dermatology.
Among other things they provide
patient information leaflets
about various skin diseases,
including psoriasis.*

British Association of Skin Camouflage
c/o Resources for Business
South Park Road
Macclesfield SK11 6SH
Tel: 01625 267880
Fax: 01625 267879
Email: thorpm@resources.demon.co.uk
A network of practitioners trained in camouflage techniques for skin conditions and disfiguring injuries.

British Homoeopathic Association
27a Devonshire Street
London W1N 1RJ
Tel: 020 7935 2163
One of two regulatory bodies of homoeopaths; members are also trained doctors. Send sae (60p) for information.

British Red Cross
9 Grosvenor Crescent
London SW1X 7EJ
Tel: 020 7201 5173
Website: www.redcross.org.uk
Offer a camouflage service using special techniques to cover up unwanted skin changes.

Citizens Advice Bureau
For a wide range of advice, including financial and state benefits. Look in the telephone directory for your local branch.

Institute for Complementary Medicine
PO Box 194
London SE16 1QZ
Tel: 020 7237 5165 (weekdays 10am–2pm)
Information and advice about complementary therapy. (Please send self-addressed envelope and two 2nd class stamps.)

Long-Term Medical Conditions Alliance
Unit 212
16 Baldwins Gardens
London EC1N 7RJ
Tel: 020 7813 3637
Fax: 020 7813 3640
Website: www.lmca.demon.co.uk
Made up of over 100 organisations, the alliance campaigns on behalf of people with long-term medical conditions. Psoriasis is represented.

Motability
Goodman House
Station Approach
Harlow
Essex CM20 2ET
Tel: 01279 635 999
Helpline: 01279 635 666
Advice and help about cars, scooters and wheelchairs for people with disabilities.

NHS Health Information Service
0800 66 55 44
For information about NHS services in your area, and waiting times for appointments/admissions. They also have details about patient support groups, conditions and possible treatments.

Primary Care Dermatology
Society
PO Box 6
Princes Risborough HP7 9XD
Tel: 01844 276271
Email: enquires@rpsgb.org.uk
Website: www.rpsgb.org.uk
An organisation made up of GPs who have a special interest in dermatology.

Skin Treatment and Research
Trust (START)
Chelsea and Westminster Hospital
369 Fulham Road
London SW10 9NH
Tel: 020 8746 8174
Primarily a laboratory research establishment, not an information service, but they may be able to give information about specific research questions.

Society of Homoeopaths
2 Artizan Road
Northampton NN1 4HU
Tel: 01604 621400
One of two regulatory bodies of homoeopaths.

Websites that we have checked out

www.tecc.co.uk/public.psoriasis/psor.html
This has not been updated recently; it is a personal account from someone with psoriasis and includes some information about treatments.

www.paalliance.org
Another British website, written by the Psoriatic Arthropathy Alliance and therefore focuses on arthropathy although there is also information about psoriasis in general. It lists information sheets that you can send for.

www/psoriasis.org/npf.shtml
This is the website of the American National Psoriasis Foundation. It is regularly updated and has a lot of very good information about research and practical advice. Do note that it is American, so some of the information about products etc. may not be relevant in Britain.

www.psoriasis.org/ifpa.html
This is an extension of the National Psoriasis Foundation, giving information about the International Federation of Psoriasis Associations. It provides contacts for different associations world-wide. Although the Psoriasis Association is not listed, the Psoriatic Arthropathy Alliance is.

Appendix 2

Useful publications

Publications for people with psoriasis

Psoriasis: a patient's guide, by N.J. Lowe, published by Martin Dunitz, London (1999)

Coping with Psoriasis, by Ronald Marks, published by Sheldon, London (1997)

Publications for health care professionals

ABC of Dermatology, 2nd edition, edited by P.K. Buxton, published by BMJ Books, London (1998)

Clinical Dermatology, by J.A.A. Hunter, J.A. Savin and M.V. Dahl, published by Blackwell Scientific Publications, Oxford (1990)

Appendix 3

Tables of products and their relative cost if bought over the counter

Table 1 Emollients

Name of product	Greasiness	Amount	Approx. cost
Aveeno bath oil	Slightly greasy	250ml	£7
Aveeno cream	Slightly greasy	100ml	£6
Balneum bath oil	Slightly greasy	200ml	£5
Dermol 500 lotion	Slightly greasy	500ml	£12
Diprobase cream	Slightly greasy	500g	£12
Diprobath bath additive	Slightly greasy	500ml	£13
E45 emollient bath oil	Slightly greasy	500ml	£7
E45 emollient wash cream	Slightly greasy	250ml	£4
E45 cream	Slightly greasy	500g	£9
E45 lotion	Hardly greasy	500ml	£6
Epaderm ointment	Very greasy	500g	£11
Oilatum emollient bath additive	Slightly greasy	250ml	£5
Oilatum shower emollient	Hardly greasy	125g	£9
Unguentum M cream	Very greasy	500g	£19

This is only a small sample of the bath oils creams, lotions and ointments available over the counter. It is important that you make sure you are using the one that suits you best and that is most effective on your skin. Your doctor will prescribe most of these, and generally it is cheaper to get them on prescription – especially if you ask for the larger sizes. The products often come in a variety of sizes, so you can get bigger or smaller versions than the ones indicated here.

Table 2 Tar-based treatments

Name of product	Amount	Approx. cost
Alphosyl cream	100g	£4
Alphosyl 2 in 1 shampoo	250ml	£6
Capasal shampoo	250ml	£8
Clinitar cream	100g	£19
Cocois scalp ointment	100g	£17
Exorex lotion	250ml	£30
Polytar liquid (shampoo)	250ml	£4
T-Gel (shampoo)	250ml	£7

Table 3 Topical steroids classified by potency

Group strength	Chemical (generic) name	Trade name
Very potent	0.05% clobetasol propionate	Dermovate
	0.3% diflucortolone valerate	Nerisone Forte
Potent	0.1% betamethasone valerate	Betnovate
	0.025% fluocinolone acetonide	Synalar
	0.1% mometasone furoate	Elocon*
	0.05% fluticasone propionate	Cutivate*
Moderately potent	0.025% betamethasone valerate	1/4 Betnovate (otherwise known as Betnovate RD)
	0.00625% fluocinolone acetonide	Synalar 1 in 4
	0.05% clobetasone butyrate	Eumovate
	0.05% alclometasone dipropionate	Modrasone
Mild	2.5% hydrocortisone	Efcortelan
	1% hydrocortisone	Dioderm

* For use only once a day.

Appendix 4

Fact sheet on psoriasis

Here are some of the important facts about psoriasis. Please feel free to photocopy this sheet and use it to inform those around you.

1. Around 2% of the UK population have psoriasis (1 in 50 people).
2. It affects men and women equally.
3. It is **not** contagious.
4. It is **not** related to poor hygiene.
5. It is thought to be passed on from one generation to another but it is possible to carry the psoriasis gene without having any signs of the disease.
6. There are several factors that are thought to trigger episodes of active psoriasis:
   - Injury to the skin – for example, a cut or graze or even rubbing from clothes – may cause psoriasis to appear at the point of the injury.
   - Shock or long-term stress can cause psoriasis to develop.
   - Certain drugs are related to the appearance of psoriasis; these include beta-blockers, anti-malarial drugs and lithium.
   - Drinking too much alcohol can aggravate psoriasis and will certainly make it feel worse.
   - Smoking is thought to make psoriasis worse, especially pustular psoriasis on the hands and feet.
7. People who get psoriasis can have periods of remission when they have no psoriasis on their skin at all.
8. Psoriasis is usually treated using creams and ointments but in severe cases drugs might be taken by mouth.

9. Many people with psoriasis find that sunlight makes their psoriasis better, but 10% find that it actually makes it worse.

10. Psoriasis can feel extremely uncomfortable (dry, itchy, sore and sometimes painful).

Index

NOTE This index covers pages 1 to 126. Page numbers followed by italic *g* indicate glossary.

The Psoriasis Association

Charity number 257414

- Founded in 1968 by Dr Dick Coles and a group of patients at Northampton, the Association has become an important self-help organisation providing support and mutual aid for sufferers.
- It is advised by an eminent Medical and Research Committee, and each year supports important research projects.
- Considerable publicity and education has increased the community understanding and acceptance of psoriasis.
- The Association continually works to raise standards of patient care through its contacts with the medical professions, the social services, government departments and other organisations.
- The Association has become the main source of information on all aspects of psoriasis.
- Close links have been formed with similar organisations throughout the world.
- The Association is managed by an elected Council of voluntary members supported by a small number of full-time employees.
- Membership is open to anyone. Every Member receives the national Journal *Psoriasis* three times a year. This includes articles by both sufferers and medical experts on all aspects of psoriasis.

Members may also participate voluntarily in the activities of their local Groups. These meet regularly to provide points of social contact and information, and to raise funds for research and educational projects.

Aims

To help people with psoriasis by

- Collecting funds for and promoting research.
- Advancing education in all aspects of the condition.
- Increasing public acceptance and understanding.
- Representing their national and local interests.
- Providing a point of social contact.

For contact details, see Appendix 1, earlier.

The Psoriatic Arthropathy Alliance

Charity number 1051169

The Psoriatic Arthropathy Alliance (PAA) is a national registered charity dedicated to raising awareness and helping people with psoriatic arthritis and its associated skin disorder psoriasis.

The organisation was co-founded by David and Julie Chandler (David has the condition) in April 1993, both being spurred on by the lack of adequate information available to patients and the general public.

Although psoriatic arthritis is considered by many to be a minority illness of the 2–3% of the UK population who have psoriasis, between 10 and 20% of these people will develop psoriatic arthritis, which makes it the second most common rheumatic arthritis in the UK.

Since the charity's launch in the Jubilee Room at the House of Commons, hosted by David Congdon, former chairman of the All Party Parliamentary Group on Skin, the PAA has continually achieved the following:

- Consistently produced publications for its members and professionals.
- Held annual national conferences.
- Developed its own Internet site.
- Undertaken a national awareness campaign with a spring 'awareness' week.
- Dealt with, on average, over 5,000 enquiries each year.
- Contributed to the debate for better healthcare for patients.
- Made links with similar organisations nationally and internationally.
- Developed a strong board of medical and non-medical advisers.

Membership is available to all and includes free back issues of all publications, information sheets, free entry to the annual conference and unique access to contacts throughout the UK.

For further information about the PAA or its activities, see the contact details in Appendix 1, earlier.

We hope you found *Psoriasis at your fingertips* interesting and helpful. If you enjoyed it, you might be interested in the following extract from *Allergies at your fingertips* by Dr Joanne Clough.

Appendix 1

Diagnosing your allergies

In this appendix my aim is to give you a description of each of the common allergy tests, including details of what you will feel and whether they are uncomfortable. I also suggest when each test may be needed, pointing out any special instructions relating to the tests, and discussing their individual advantages and disadvantages. I hope this information will help you to understand why your doctor has chosen one test rather than another. I also briefly describe a number of tests sometimes used by practitioners of complementary techniques, although few of these are felt to have a place in the diagnosis of allergy.

Why test?

If you have had an allergic reaction and its cause is uncertain or unknown, you will need to have one or more of the tests described here. Even if you know the cause of your allergic reaction, you may still need to have the diagnosis confirmed by some form of allergy testing, particularly if you have had a severe allergic reaction, or if you have multiple allergies, or if your doctor is considering any form of treatment that is going to be long-lasting, difficult, time-consuming or expensive. If you are going to help with the evaluation of a new treatment, you will certainly need to have your allergy confirmed by formal testing. If there is any confusion as to whether your problem is caused by a true allergy (i.e. one involving the production of the allergy antibody IgE, as discussed in the section *Allergy explained* in Chapter 1) or some other process is involved, allergy testing can clear up this doubt. Finally, if having an allergy has any legal implications for you (e.g. if you might be eligible for compensation), the diagnosis must be confirmed by appropriate tests.

Each year 10% of the population of the UK experience an allergic problem of some kind, and 25% of the population will, during their lifetimes, see a doctor because of an allergy. As these problems are now so common, allergy testing is being carried out more often and is becoming increasingly sophisticated. However, there is no point in doing allergy tests if either you or your doctor is going to be unwilling to take action based on the results. If a true allergy is diagnosed, you may benefit not only from medications aimed at treating the allergic reaction once it has happened but also from preventive action, both in the form of drugs and in the form of allergen avoidance.

Choosing the most suitable test

Different allergies are more common at different ages, and so the type of allergy test you will be offered by your doctor depends, to some extent, on your age. Food allergies are more common in infancy and early childhood, whereas problems caused by allergens in the air become more common after the age of 5 years. Allergies to insect stings usually start in adulthood, and can be particularly troublesome in older people.

Every test performed in the diagnosis of allergies should be:

- relevant (there is no point in doing skin prick testing or patch testing unless you include the likely culprits);
- standardised (so that the result of a test done in one hospital means the same as that done in a different hospital);
- repeatable (so that the results on one occasion can be compared with the results of the same test on a different occasion);
- specific (so that the test is positive only in people who have that allergy); and
- sensitive (so that the test is negative only in people who do not have the problem).

This is a lot to ask of any test, and it is impossible for any one test to score 100% on all of these points. Every test has its advantages and its disadvantages, and this is why specialist knowledge is necessary to make sure that the right test is chosen for you.

By far the most useful information available to your doctor will come from your medical history – the account that you give of your allergic reaction and your answers to a large number of questions, including:

- your general status (age, job, and so on);
- any illnesses you have had in the past;
- whether there are other members of your family with allergic problems;
- the details of your own allergic problems; and
- how often you are exposed to allergens and to other factors that can make allergic problems worse (e.g. cigarette smoke, air pollution and certain drugs).

All of these details must be taken into account when assessing the result of any allergy test. If your allergy is particularly troublesome or if you have had a severe allergic reaction, it is advisable that you be referred to an allergy specialist.

Skin prick testing

Description

This is probably the most commonly used allergy test. It is performed on the skin of your back or of your inner forearm, and you can be tested to up to 25 allergens at any one time. A drop of the allergen extract is placed on your skin, which is pricked through the drop using a lancet (a small sharp prong just 1mm long). A positive result consists of a weal (a pale bump) which may be itchy and surrounded by a red area or 'flare'. The size of the weal is measured after 10 minutes, and any weal of greater than 2mm (or, in some cases, 3mm) in size is regarded as being positive.

Two additional substances will always be included in this form of testing: a positive and a negative control. The positive control solution contains histamine, to which everyone should react. Failure to do so can result from treatment with certain medicines (including antihistamines, corticosteroids and certain antidepressant drugs) and will alert the tester to the fact that the results of testing will be unreliable. The negative control is made from a saline solution, to which no one should react. A positive reaction to this negative control shows that the skin is, for some reason, extremely sensitive, and once again indicates that testing will not be reliable.

Skin prick testing is a painless procedure, which is well tolerated even by small infants. Positive reactions may be somewhat itchy, but this will subside within an hour.

Skin prick testing is a very sensitive diagnostic tool, but not everyone who has a positive test has symptoms of an allergy. If you do not develop a reaction to an allergen, you can be almost certain that you are not allergic to it. However, a positive reaction may be highlighting a hidden or latent allergy that is not currently causing you problems, but that might show up later on in your life.

Indications
Skin prick testing is usually the first test recommended when an allergy is suspected.

Special instructions
Tell the person doing the skin prick testing if you are on any medication. If it is safe to do so, treatment with antihistamines, corticosteroids or tricyclic antidepressants should be stopped for an appropriate time (up to two weeks) before the test is carried out. However, these medications should be stopped only on your doctor's instructions.

Advantages
This is a simple, quick and inexpensive form of testing, which can be performed to a very wide range of different allergens. It can give useful information in all forms of allergy, and provides results within 15 minutes.

Disadvantages
Skin prick testing is unreliable in the very young and older people. It cannot be performed if you are taking certain medication (listed earlier in this section) or in people with severe eczema. Although generally extremely safe, skin prick testing may provoke a severe allergic reaction in people who have previously experienced anaphylaxis (discussed in Chapter 6), although this is extremely rare.

Intradermal testing

Description
Intradermal literally means 'within the skin', from the Latin word 'intra' meaning 'within' and the Greek word 'derma' meaning 'skin'. In this test a small amount of a diluted allergen extract is injected beneath the surface of your skin. A reaction is usually apparent within 10–20 minutes, and takes the form of swelling, itching and a raised weal (a pale bump).

This form of testing is now rarely used in the UK, as not only does it give inaccurate results (using a high concentration of allergen can falsely indicate allergy where none exists) but also it can be dangerous, with a higher risk of anaphylactic reactions (anaphylaxis is discussed in Chapter 6).

Patch testing

Description
For this test allergens are prepared in appropriate concentrations in white soft paraffin (e.g. Vaseline) and are then spread onto discs the size of a one pence piece. The discs (made of a special metal that cannot itself provoke a reaction) are placed on your skin (usually on your back) and covered with an adhesive dressing. They are left in place for 48 hours, after which your skin is examined, and any redness and swelling are noted. Your skin will be re-examined after a further 48 hours for any remaining redness or swelling. The interpretation of this form of testing is not as simple as it sounds, and should be done only by someone with skill and experience.

Indications
Patch testing is performed in cases of contact dermatitis where allergy is suspected.

Special instructions
The symptoms of contact dermatitis must be brought under control using an appropriate steroid cream before patch testing can be carried out, or else the results will be unreliable. These steroid creams should then be discontinued for at least 3–4 weeks before testing, as they may suppress the test response.

Advantages
This is a relatively simple, safe and inexpensive form of testing, which is particularly useful for all forms of contact dermatitis.

Disadvantages
Interpretation of the results is not easy, and requires a thorough knowledge of your allergy history and of the materials in question. Almost 10% of the normal healthy population with no skin disease will demonstrate unexpected, apparently irrelevant, positive results. Itching or blistering may develop as a response to the test allergens.

Radioallergosorbent test (RAST)

Description
This is a blood test that measures the amount of specific IgE your immune system has produced against a suspected allergen. For example, if you have asthma, it can confirm that you have antibodies against the house dust mite. (There is more information about IgE and other antibodies in the section *Allergy explained* in Chapter 1.)

The test is carried out on a small sample of blood, which is taken from a vein in your arm using a fine needle and a small syringe. Although some people dislike needles, the blood test causes minimal discomfort. The sample is then sent to a specialist laboratory, and the results are available within a few days.

RAST uses a technique in which a radioactive 'label' is allowed to attach itself to the IgE present in your blood sample. Measuring the amount of radioactivity left at the completion of the test provides information about any specific antibodies you have produced. The total amount of IgE in your bloodstream is usually measured at the same time, so that the amount of any specific IgE which is found can be compared to the total amount in your blood.

Indications
This test is increasing in popularity, and is often used in conjunction with skin prick testing. It is particularly useful when the risk of an anaphylactic reaction (discussed in Chapter 6) makes skin prick testing too risky; when extensive eczema makes skin prick testing impractical; and when allergic symptoms are so severe that antihistamine medication cannot be discontinued to permit accurate skin prick testing.

Special instructions
Local anaesthetic cream may be available for small children and for adults who particularly request it, to eliminate any discomfort from blood sampling. This cream takes an hour to be effective, so must be applied and covered by an adhesive dressing before the test.

Advantages
This form of allergy testing is completely safe. It is specific, in that if a RAST is positive it is likely that you have a true allergy, but false negative results can occur.

Disadvantages
The test involves taking a sample of blood, which some people find unpleasant. It is expensive. A negative result does not completely rule out the possibility that allergy to that allergen exists. Do not assume that you are not at risk from a particular allergen just because the RAST is negative.

Other blood tests

Multiple RAST

A form of RAST that can test for several allergens at once is now available, and is being marketed commercially through a number of large supermarkets. Because this form of testing can yield positive results when no allergy is present (false positives), as well as giving negative results when an allergy does in fact exist (false negatives), it should not be performed without the results being put in the context of a full medical history and interpreted by a trained doctor.

Other antibody tests

Although most allergy testing involves looking for evidence of the IgE antibody, in some circumstances (such as coeliac disease, discussed in Chapter 5) evidence of other antibodies such as IgA or IgG is helpful in making a diagnosis. (There is more information about these antibodies in the section *Allergy explained* in Chapter 1.) As far as you are concerned, the test simply involves giving a blood sample as you would for RAST (as described in the previous section of this appendix).

Challenge tests

Sometimes the only way to confirm an allergy is deliberately to provoke the symptoms it causes. Challenge tests (also called provocation tests) can also be used to demonstrate that a particular allergen is *not* responsible for your symptoms.

Airways challenge tests

Description

You inhale increasing concentrations of either a histamine-like substance or of a specific allergen solution made from the substance suspected of causing your asthma or hayfever symptoms. Your response to each dose is measured using lung function tests (described later in this appendix). The test is continued until there is a predetermined drop in your lung function. At this point, your chest may feel a little tight and you may be a little wheezy, but these symptoms will be mild. Your lung function is then returned to normal by giving you a bronchodilator (reliever) inhaler to use (these inhalers are discussed in the section *Treatment* in Chapter 2).

Indications

This form of testing is rarely used, but it can be particularly useful in the diagnosis of asthma brought on by substances encountered in the workplace. It is also used in allergy research.

Special instructions

Bronchodilator medications and drinks containing caffeine must be avoided for at least four hours before testing, and you must be free from colds.

Advantages

This form of testing can be very useful when it is helpful for your doctor to have a measurable or quantifiable response; for example, to find out if one drug suits you better than another, or to see if someone's asthma gets better when he or she stops working with a particular chemical.

Disadvantages

Although it is not painful, this procedure can be rather intimidating because of the equipment used, and requires a high degree of co-operation from the person being tested. Because of this, it cannot usually be performed on children under 7 years old. If an allergen is used, you will be kept under observation for at least eight hours after the test. There is a small risk of a severe asthma reaction, so this form of testing will only be performed by an experienced practitioner who has the facilities available to handle emergencies. These tests are relatively time-consuming and therefore expensive.

Oral challenge tests (food challenges)

Description
The food or foods suspected of causing allergic reactions are eliminated completely from your diet. If your symptoms disappear, these foods are reintroduced one at a time, at intervals of at least three days, to see if your symptoms recur. To make sure that your ideas on what causes your symptoms cannot bias the results, foods are often reintroduced in capsule form so that you don't know which food is which (this is called a single blind challenge). Even better is the form of challenge in which neither you nor your doctor knows which food is being reintroduced (a double blind challenge). In a double blind challenge, someone who is not involved with the testing process keeps the records.

Indications
This form of testing can be useful when food allergy has been previously diagnosed using inappropriate or invalid tests; when your symptoms are not typical of an allergy but may be due to some form of food intolerance; or when several skin prick test results are positive and it is unclear which of the foods tested is causing your symptoms.

Special instructions
This form of testing should never be performed on anyone who has suffered an anaphylactic reaction due to food allergy (anaphylaxis is discussed in Chapter 6).

Advantages
Double blind food challenge is extremely reliable, and if an allergy is present, symptoms will appear when the food responsible is introduced. If no symptoms occur, allergy can be ruled out.

Disadvantages
There is a risk of severe allergic or anaphylactic reactions, so this form of testing should only be carried out in a hospital by expert and

experienced medical staff who are fully trained and equipped to handle emergencies.

Lung function testing

Two forms of lung function test are commonly used in the diagnosis of asthma, both of which simply involve you blowing out air as hard and as fast as you can into the mouthpiece of a piece of equipment. Full lung spirometry (which measures how quickly and efficiently you can empty your lungs) is generally only carried out in a hospital, as the equipment required is relatively expensive, although some GPs now have this facility. Peak expiratory flow testing, which is described here, is more commonly used as you can do it at home.

Peak expiratory flow testing

Description
This test is also known as peak flow testing or peak flow monitoring. It uses a peak expiratory flow meter (more usually called a peak flow meter), which is a small hand-held device that measures how fast air can be blown out from your lungs. If you have asthma, not only will your readings be lower than those of people without asthma who are of your age, height and gender (all things that affect the readings), but your readings will also be more variable from day to day. One-off readings are therefore not particularly helpful, so you will usually be given your own meter and asked to keep twice-daily recordings on a special chart, recording the best of three readings each time.

To make a reading, you take a full deep breath in, you place the instrument between your lips so that an airtight seal is made between your lips and the mouthpiece, and you then blow through the device as hard and as fast as you can. Air passing through the meter moves a small pointer across a scale, indicating the maximum flow achieved. The pointer must be reset before each blow.

Indications
Peak flow recordings can be useful in the following situations:

- to diagnose asthma;
- to judge whether a treatment is leading to improvement;
- to help judge the need for increased treatment if your asthma is going out of control;

- if you find it difficult to judge how bad your asthma is;
- in asthma research.

Special instructions
You should have your own device, as readings can vary slightly between meters. The device should be cleaned regularly according to the manufacturer's instructions. You should be taught how to use the meter correctly, and your technique should be reviewed regularly by your doctor or practice nurse.

Advantages
Peak flow meters are relatively inexpensive, and can provide information that can be extremely helpful in the day-to-day management of asthma. For example, you and your doctor can agree on a self-management plan, which will allow you to use your peak flow readings to judge the amount of treatment you require, and to take steps to deal with any changes in your symptoms without the need to call for medical help each time.

Disadvantages
Peak flow recordings should not be used as the sole indicator of how good or bad your lungs are on any particular day – the meters are not infallible, so you should also take note of how your chest feels and what symptoms you are experiencing. It is possible to cheat with a peak flow meter, producing both falsely high and falsely low recordings.

Symptom diaries

Description
Your doctor may ask you to keep a record both of your symptoms and of the factors thought to be causing them; for example, a record of your bowel symptoms together with a list of all the foods you have eaten. Sometimes special forms are provided, but an ordinary notebook will do.

Indications
A symptom diary can be an invaluable source of information in almost any allergic problem.

Special instructions
Your doctor will explain to you exactly what is required, but you should feel free to include any extra information that you think might be helpful.

Advantages
People who suffer from allergic problems are often completely well on the days they see their doctors. It is therefore extremely useful to be able to take with you a record of how frequent and how serious your problem is, what form it takes and what might be provoking it.

Disadvantages
Not only is a symptom diary subjective, it also requires you – if it is to be of any use – to be totally honest and comprehensive when recording your exposure to allergens and any possible resulting symptoms. It may take many weeks to record enough details to provide useful information and this can require considerable effort on your part. Symptom diaries can also be difficult to interpret.

Bowel biopsy

Description
In order to diagnose coeliac disease, a bowel biopsy is necessary, and there are two ways in which this can be done. The method chosen will depend on which technique is preferred at the hospital you attend. Both methods provide a small piece of bowel lining to be examined under a microscope.

The first method uses an instrument called a gastroscope, which is a flexible tube-like viewing instrument that uses fibre optics to allow the doctor to see the inside of your digestive system. The gastroscope is inserted into your stomach or small intestine through your mouth, and a small amount of the bowel lining is taken once the instrument is in the correct position. This technique is generally used in adults.

The second method involves a small (less than 1 cm long) capsule called a Crosby capsule, which is attached to a very fine hollow tube. Again this is passed into the intestine via the mouth. Once it is in the correct position (confirmed by an X-ray), the capsule is triggered to take a small amount of the bowel lining, and then gently withdrawn. This technique is more commonly used in children.

Although both these procedures sound rather unpleasant, they are not actually as disagreeable as they seem. They are usually tolerated well, even by very small children. You will be given a sedative to help you relax while the test is being carried out. It is essential that coeliac disease is diagnosed accurately using one of these biopsy techniques, as the treatment involves lifelong avoidance of all foods containing gluten. This strict diet is not something that you would want to have to follow unnecessarily.

Environmental testing

This is a test on your surroundings, not on you. A number of substances found in the environment – both at home and at work – can cause allergic problems. Occasionally it is helpful to send samples of dust, air or chemical substances used at work for analysis. This type of testing can only be done by a specialist allergy centre.

Other tests

Alternative allergy specialists often use diagnostic tests other than the ones I have described above, and these can include the following.

Applied kinesiology

This measures muscle strength before and after exposure to a suspected allergen.

Auricular cardiac reflex method

Close proximity to a substance to which a person is allergic is said to result in a change in position in the strongest pulse at the wrist.

Hair analysis

The subject's hair is examined and medical problems are diagnosed from the appearance and content of the hair.

Leukocytotoxic tests

White blood cells are put into contact with the suspected allergen and the cells are observed under a microscope for changes in size and shape. These changes are regarded as an indication of the cells' reactivity.

Neutralisation-provocation testing (the Miller technique)

The dose of an allergen which can switch off or neutralise the allergy is found, and this dose is administered as drops under the subject's tongue.

Vega testing

This measures the electromagnetic fields produced by the subject, using a Vegatest machine.

These tests are not felt by conventional medical practitioners to be relevant, standardised or repeatable, and are considered to have no place in the diagnosis of true allergy.

Have you found **Psoriasis at your fingertips** practical and useful? If so, you may be interested in other books from Class Publishing.

Allergies at your fingertips
£14.99
Dr Joanne Clough

At last – sensible practical advice on allergies from an experienced medical expert.

'An excellent book which deserves to be on the bookshelf of every family.'
Dr Csaba Rusznak, Medical and Scientific Director, British Allergy Foundation

Asthma at your fingertips
NEW THIRD EDITION!   £14.99
Dr Mark Levy, Professor Sean Hilton and Greta Barnes MBE

This book shows you how to keep your asthma – or your family's asthma – under control, making it easier to live a full, happy and healthy life.

'This book gives you the knowledge. Don't limit yourself.'
Adrian Moorhouse MBE, Olympic Gold Medallist

High blood pressure at your fingertips
NEW SECOND EDITION!   £14.99
Dr Julian Tudor Hart with Dr Tom Fahey

The authors use all their years of experience as blood pressure experts to answer your questions on high blood pressure.

'Readable and comprehensive information.'
Dr Sylvia McLaughlan, Director General, The Stroke Association

Diabetes at your fingertips
£14.99
Professor Peter Sonksen, Dr Charles Fox and Sister Sue Judd

461 questions on diabetes are answered clearly and accurately – the ideal reference book for everyone with diabetes.

'I have no hesitation in commending this book.'
Sir Harry Secombe CBE, President of the British Diabetic Association

Stop that heart attack!
£14.99
Dr Derrick Cutting

The easy, drug-free and medically accurate way to cut dramatically your risk of having a heart attack.

Even if you already have heart disease, you can halt and even reverse its progress by following Dr Cutting's simple steps. Don't be a victim – take action NOW!

Heart health at your fingertips
£14.99
Dr Graham Jackson

This practical handbook, written by a leading cardiologist, answers all your questions about heart conditions.

'Contains the answers the doctor wishes he had given if only he'd had time.'
Dr Thomas Stuttaford, The Times

Eczema and your child
£11.99
Dr Tim Mitchell, Dr David Paige and Karen Spowart

This practical and medically accurate handbook will guide you through the maze of old wives' tales, unscientific advice and outdated treatments.

'It addresses the questions we are asked all the time.'
Mercy Jeyasingham, Director of Education and Information, National Eczema Society

Parkinson's at your fingertips
NEW SECOND EDITION!   £14.99
Dr Marie Oxtoby and Professor Adrian Williams

Full of practical help and advice for people with Parkinson's disease and their families. This book gives you the information and the confidence to tackle the challenges that PD presents.

> 'An unqualified success.'
> Dr Andrew Lees, Consultant Neurologist,
> The National Hospital for Neurology and Neurosurgery

Cancer information at your fingertips
£14.99
Val Speechley and Maxine Rosenfield

Recommended by the Cancer Research Campaign, this book provides straightforward and positive answers to all your questions about cancer.

Stroke at your fingertips
NEW!   £14.99
Dr Anthony Rudd, Penny Irwin SRN and Bridget Penhale

This essential guidebook tells you all about strokes – most importantly how to recover from them.

Full of practical advice, and including recuperation plans, you will find this book invaluable.

Alzheimer's at your fingertips
£14.99
Harry Cayton, Dr Nori Graham and Dr James Warner

At last – a book that tells you everything you need to know about Alzheimer's and other dementias.

> 'an invaluable contribution to understanding all forms of dementia'
> Dr Jonathan Miller CBE,
> President, Alzheimer's Disease Society

Epilepsy at your fingertips
£14.99
Brian Chappell and Professor Pamela Crawford

The authors answer over 220 real questions from people with epilepsy – giving you the knowledge to lead an active and fulfilled life!

Multiple sclerosis at your fingertips
NEW!   £14.99
Ian Robinson, Dr Stuart Neilson and Dr Frank Clifford Rose

The expert authors pass on all the useful, practical information they have learnt over the years. There is specific information on areas such as driving, holidays, work, children, sexual relationships and other people's attitudes

> 'an invaluable resource'
> Jan Hatch, Director of MS Services,
> MS Society

Your child's epilepsy: a parent's guide
£11.99
Dr Richard Appleton, Brian Chappell and Margaret Beirne

If your child has epilepsy, you will find this practical guide invaluable. It answers the questions you really want to ask, from diagnosis to treatment and from schools to relationships.

Kidney failure explained
NEW!   £14.99
Dr Andy Stein and Janet Wild

Everything you always wanted to know about kidney failure but were afraid to ask!

PRIORITY ORDER FORM

Cut out or photocopy this form and send it (post free in the UK) to:

Class Publishing Priority Service   Tel: 01752 202301
FREEPOST (no stamp needed)
London W6 7BR   Fax: 01752 202333

Please send me urgently   **Post included**
(*tick boxes below*)   **price per copy**
                                                     (*UK only*)

- ☐ **Psoriasis at your fingertips** (ISBN 1 872362 99 0)   £17.99
- ☐ **Allergies at your fingertips** (ISBN 1 872362 52 4)   £17.99
- ☐ **Asthma at your fingertips** (ISBN 1 872362 006 3)   £17.99
- ☐ **High blood pressure at your fingertips** (ISBN 1 872362 99 0) £17.99
- ☐ **Diabetes at your fingertips** (ISBN 1 872362 79 6)   £17.99
- ☐ **Stop that heart attack** (ISBN 1 872362 85 0)   £17.99
- ☐ **Heart health at your fingertips** (ISBN 1 872362 77 X)   £17.99
- ☐ **Eczema and your child** (ISBN 1 872362 86 9)   £14.99
- ☐ **Parkinson's at your fingertips** (ISBN 1 872362 96 6)   £17.99
- ☐ **Cancer information at your fingertips** (ISBN 1 872362 56 7)   £17.99
- ☐ **Stroke at your fingertips** (ISBN 1 872362 98 2)   £17.99
- ☐ **Alzheimer's at your fingertips** (ISBN 1 872362 71 0)   £17.99
- ☐ **Epilepsy at your fingertips** (ISBN 1 872362 51 6)   £17.99
- ☐ **Multiple sclerosis at your fingertips** (ISBN 1 872362 94 X)   £17.99
- ☐ **Your child's epilepsy** (ISBN 1 872362 61 3)   £14.99
- ☐ **Kidney failure explained** (ISBN 1 872362 90 7)   £17.99

TOTAL: _____

Easy ways to pay

Cheque: I enclose a cheque payable to Class Publishing for £_____

Credit card: please debit my ☐ Access ☐ Visa ☐ Amex ☐ Switch

Number: ☐☐☐☐☐☐☐☐☐☐☐☐☐☐☐☐☐   Expiry date:

Name _____

My address for delivery is _____

_____

Town _____ County _____ Postcode _____

Telephone number (*in case of query*) _____

Credit card billing address if different from above _____

_____

Town _____ County _____ Postcode _____

Class Publishing's guarantee: remember that if, for any reason, you are not satisfied with these books, we will refund all your money, without any questions asked. Prices and VAT rates may be altered for reasons beyond our control.